GAME
Of
HEALTH

By
Tim Sologhashvili

Copyright page

Copyright © 2019 by BAEMS All rights reserved. This book or any portion thereof may not be reproduced or used in any manner whatsoever without the express written permission of the publisher. Except for the use of brief quotations in a book review.

TABLE OF CONTENTS

THE PREFACE 4
INTRODUCTION 5
CHAPTER I GAME 5-0-1 12
CHAPTER II BORING 16
CHAPTER III TIME 20
CHAPTER IV STRESS 23
CHAPTER V GYM NONSENSE 33
CHAPTER VI GO ORGANIC 35
CHAPTER VII GREEN PAGES 40
CHAPTER VIII YELLOW PAGES 77
CHAPTER IX RED PAGES 90
CHAPTER X REUSABLE PLASTIC CUPS AND FOOD CONTAINERS 102
CHAPTER XI MINDFULNESS 108
CHAPTER XII MEDITATION 112
CHAPTER XIII YOGA 114
CHAPTER XIV EASY & HEALTHY RECIPES 119
CHAPTER XV THE RAW FOOD DIET 131
CHAPTER XVI FOODS THAT BENEFIT VARIOUS BODY PARTS 134
CHAPTER XVII ESSENTIAL VITAMINS AND MINERALS 138
AESTHETICS 159

THE PREFACE

It took me a long to discover the truth. On the journey, I have chased fame and money because I thought it was an answer to true happiness and joy. I tried to exercise a lot to have a perfect body because I thought girls love guys in good shape. Every time I manage to achieve one goal, I discovered something was still missing. Finally, I found an answer, and I would like to share it with you now. These are tips for physical and mental health, and these tips should lead you on the right path. I talk about the benefits of nutrition, meditation, mindfulness, and yoga because I believe all these things are essential for living a happy and healthy life. I also talk about what is extremely bad for our health, such as sugar, plastic, and so on. We need to know how each food affects our body and how much to eat. Eating healthy is not enough. We also need to understand how to save energy. We are continuously thinking, most of the time, nonsense. So we drain up our strength. That's why we need to practice meditation and mindfulness. In general, eating and drinking shouldn't be our concern at all, but unfortunately, it is today for most of us. As one great Greek philosopher Socrates once said: "Worthless people live only to eat and drink; people of worth eat and drink only to live."

INTRODUCTION

Since I was a very young kid, I've always been into sports. I attended judo classes: not because I loved it, but because there was just one sport in my town and it was free! During those afternoons, I learned a lot about sparring and not a thing about nutrition. I was doing ok, though if only I knew more about how food affects the majority of one's body and mind, I could have done way better, reaching the very top and the best version of myself. I could have used my entire potential, instead of only 30-40% of it.

Overall, we had a good time sparring and playing, but I'm not going to talk about my past now, I'm not going to waste your time with useless stories. No, this is my own experience and research about how to be in good shape and how to keep it precisely this way throughout our lives.

No matter how old, how big or how small you are, anyone can do it; here is an essential message: we need to trust ourselves and be driven by the motivation to unleash our untapped inner power. We have to do it by staying true to ourselves and our goal: no cheating, no breaking the rules!

I used a little trick to remind myself to stay focused and motivated during the change until the time my body accepted the new nutritional lifestyle as being the best and most natural. I had a little piece of paper on which I had jotted down my commitment: "I do believe in myself," followed by a line saying that I will not break the rules for my good! You could even take a picture of that valuable note and make it a background image on your phone as a great reminder. Committing is very important. No rules = no game and no game = no gain, it's that simple. In our lives we all play some game by some standards, some of us are winners, some losers, but if you never play you can never win. So test yourself and be ready to fight for it. I hope my words will guide you to shine. You don't have to win all the games, because, I tell you, not all the games are your games, but you don't want to miss your chance at your game, you don't want to be one of those people for whom life happens passively without ever playing their game. They are not playing, yet somehow they do go a great deal to convince themselves that they still could win something. Believe it or not, sadly, they can never win.

Do you want to have a beautiful body? Good health? Do you want to be financially independent? Set your game, play by it, and be patient, don't listen to cheap advice, there are plenty of people around us who have done nothing for themselves, yet they'll tell you what to do, how to train, what to eat. Don't listen to shallow preachers.

Pick the right book for you; there are plenty of books to read! I read hundreds of them and more. Some were boring, some were great, but the point is never giving up on your search for the knowledge that will unlock the best possible version of yourself. If you make an unlucky pick, don't give up! Read another one, learn, take the right strategies, and apply them to your life.

Change your life. Make it yours, write down your own rules and play your game. Even if you don't get results at the beginning, that's ok; the most important thing is that you keep trying. The more you try, the sooner you'll succeed. But what is it, this game I'm talking?

In short, anything and everything you do is a game; life is a game! When you are born, you start playing! Then some of us are more disciplined, we play and struggle more, and in the end, we are more successful than others. Some are too lazy.

The truth is simple.

Do you want to have complete control over your body? To be in good shape, go to the gym, to the park, exercise, keep count of how much fat, sugar, and calories you are consuming every day: that becomes your game.

Your will is powerful.

Do you want to be rich? Start a business! As an employee you would never get rich because you are playing the employers' game, no matter who your employer is, whether it is the government or a private entrepreneur, it is their game you are playing. They are the ones who win or lose. But you? You are not getting your chance, you cannot succeed, and you cannot fail, you will be there to get your cut, the salary they'll determine shall be given to you for your time, knowledge and experience. So you'll be eking it out throughout your life in exchange for your time because this is really in exchange for your soul. Time is limited, and the most precious thing we have, yet we are allowing ourselves to be enslaved to someone in exchange for money, a payment that can never be fair. We are doing something we don't like, very often even hating doing it, but we still put our soul down in exchange for passive survival.

Just think about it!

If I offered you five years of the salary you make at your current job, all at once, adding the bonuses and increases you may expect in exchange for five years of your lifetime on Earth, would you sell them to me? Let's say you make £20,000 a year; we'll add some bonuses and pretend I'd give you the £120, 000 you need, tax-free. You won't waste your time for the morning and evening commute; you won't spend 8-10 hours a day, five days a week, wearing a uniform you hate and being held captive in a building you see more than your own home. Every day of every week of the next five years, none of this nonsense, you are just free. All you have to do is give up five years of your life, five years you will never get back, for a very satisfying immediate prize. My question is: would you do it? Would you sell it? Most likely, you will not! Unless you have lost a desire for life! If your answer is no, which is very logical indeed, then why do you sell your breath away, day by day, for much less than I'm offering? Consider paying no taxes, wearing no uniform, no travel card and daily expenses at work, not starting your day smelling the breath of the person standing next to you, and being way too close in a train with people packed like sardines, where personal space is only a distant memory, and the ride is overpriced and never on time.

We always have excuses, we tell ourselves many times "maybe tomorrow," "I don't have money," "it's not the right moment," "I'm not ready," and so on. The thing is when the time comes, and you finally think you are ready, sometimes it's too late.

When would you know you are ready?

You don't feel comfortable in your body, and you know that you should go for a run, join the gym, reduce your calories intake, but somehow you keep procrastinating, rescheduling your move to the next month, or telling yourself you'll do something about it after you have changed your job, or maybe after your best friend's birthday party. When the chosen day arrives, you'll have already forgotten about it, or you'll want to reschedule again! Why do we do that? Because it's easier. Postponing today's job is easy, not having to do any hard work at this very moment; relaxation is what we crave.

Have you ever wondered why those banks earn so much money? One of the reasons is that most customers don't pay their loans on time, even when they could, but they prefer to spend the money on something else to have immediate gratification, even if that will come at a high price later.

"Let's enjoy life now, we'll pay later, it's easy": that's what the whole social system exactly wants you to do, to keep itself thriving in spite of your dreams and desires, advertising your own enslavement to the world and calling it "self-growth", "a career", or some other sweet-sounding epithet made to blow smoke in the eyes of your instinct for real success, as well as your desire to live free and relax for a good, profound and gratifying life.

The economic system is feeding you, bombarding you continuously with cunning messages aiming to teach you to prefer instant shallow gratification over real success in life. And it's doing very well, indeed. So to go back to our example, people keep being late at paying back their loans, taking up missed payment penalties and higher loan rates all just to feel free from their duties for a little longer, all for only a short moment of glory on the due date, postponing their return to slavery for just some more time, underestimating that they'll have it way worse later on.

Living in the moment doesn't always work.

What works is setting goals for yourself and having a project for your own game, then sticking to it as if it's life or death. It is a matter of living or not living in the end.

Here I'm sharing my game with you.

Before we start, let me tell you about a rule:

RULE 1: scores are tallied weekly, not daily.

RULE 2: Never give up. If you miss one day or fail a week, it doesn't mean you are a loser! Let's say you eat and drink 1+1 during the week; you can still catch up by doing 0+1+0. But what are these numbers? One is a day during the week when you can eat and drink anything you want, and +1 will mean that you had another day when you ate and drank whatever you wanted. So what's 0? 0 stands for a day in the week when you eat salad and vegetables, so +0 will be an extra vegetable day during the same week. You'll only do +0 if you couldn't avoid +1 before. In case you reach 1+1+1, this week's game is lost. You can still minimize the loss by doing 0+0 but do not try to catch up the lost week by doing 0+0+0, because then your body will struggle and your balance will be lost, meaning that staying in the game will then be extremely difficult. Remember you will not win every game, and you don't have to. But you should win most. You plan to win the champions league, and the league championship is not played in one week, but over weeks and months. It's possible for a team to have a bad day and to lose that match, but it is the team that doesn't give up and scores the most points that win the league.

RULE 3: Memorize some of the most common harmful and healthier foods on the red, yellow, and green pages in this book. Feel free to make your green, yellow, or red sheets, and add anything extra that you know it is either good or bad to consume.

Do your research, do not just assume and certainly do not take account of what your friends are saying! Do your research.

RULE 4: Do not cheat. You are cheating yourself.

RULE 5: Don't listen to your friends, colleagues, or anyone. Stick to the plan.

CHAPTER I
GAME 5-0-1

♦♦♦

The game 5-0-1 is for those who want to get rid of extra body fat and gain lean muscles. Here is how it works: for five days of the week, you will eat low fat, low carb, and high protein food. If you have, let's say 5kg of extra body weight according to your sex, age, and measurements (you can find free calculators on Google to calculate how many calories needed a day), you need to cut 500 calories from your daily required caloric intake, so over 5 days you will consume 2500 fewer calories. At the same time, you should exercise at least 2 to 3 times a week. It's totally up to you how you want to exercise; you can go to the gym or run in the park.

0 is a green day; you should only eat vegetables.

One is a red day when you can eat and drink anything you like. You can mix 5-0-1 up however it is most convenient to you, but remember let's say you have already enjoyed one red day and something came up like someone's birthday or wedding, in this case, I wouldn't suggest you abstain and stick to the plan. No, you should take full advantage of an occasion like this and enjoy yourself. The happier you are, the easier it is to achieve long term goals, and this is a long-term goal, indeed. I have met people who say no to everyone and everything just because they have a diet plan, and they want to stick to it. They wait an entire month and give up because they are stressed out. The idea is to be happy and enjoy it. Thousands of people join a gym regularly, some of them try to go five days a week, some 3 or 4. Some have a schedule and know what to do and how to do it. Some do whatever, many of them do nothing at all, wasting gym space, sitting down, and using their smartphone. Most of them have something in common; they drink a protein shake as soon as they leave the gym. None of this matters, and of course, mobile users are complete losers as time and space wasters. I hope some of those people come across this message and stop being losers.

Stop using the cell phone when it's unnecessary to do so and do your job; being a gym member is cool for those who are getting results. But on the other hand, those who are doing everything almost correctly but fail to count calories will also lose. You will not get results. It's like 99% of us working 5 to 6 days or even seven days a week, but we are still poor. We are still in the rat race. That's because we don't calculate income and expenditures. Counting is boring. But trust me, if you want to be financially independent, you should start counting. If you're going to be in great shape, keep track of the calories, sugar, and fat you consume.

Let's make it clear once again when I say count calories; we must count. Don't just assume that you know roughly. Maybe you think you eat healthily, oatmeal in the morning with some nuts, jam or honey, then some chicken breast, salad, and some chocolate, but not much coffee. So, what is the problem here? The problem is that even if you eat healthily, you still need to count how much calories you consume a day. Have you ever experienced when you go shopping, you pick up some inexpensive items, but when you go to checkout you are surprised by how much you have to pay? You stare at the receipt and wonder why the cashier charged you so much? Maybe they made a mistake? But no, in most cases they don't make mistakes, we do! One pound, 2 pounds, zero points seventy pence, and a full basket like this will cost a surprising amount of money. It's the same scenario when you are eating little amounts all day, which will accumulate into a considerable number of calories too, transforming into fat. You know there are 364 calories in 100g of oatmeal. To burn 364 calories, you need to run at least 30 minutes. If you don't know how much oats you have in your bowl, especially if you add nuts, jam, or anything of the like, you will quickly end up eating 600-700 calories. The same goes for chicken breast or any other food except raw salads. If you don't control how much you eat, you are in trouble. You have to decide what it is that you want.

Do you want to have a lean body, great figure, and feel happy in your body? Do you want to be confident and enjoy every day, or do you want to enjoy the peace of chocolate and cookies? The joy of any cookies and chocolates will last as long as it is in your mouth, leaving you heavy and lazy all day. Do you want to be fat? To be uncomfortable in your own body? When you live in a body that you don't like and are too lazy to take action, you become ignorant. If girls or guys display no sexual attraction towards, don't look at you, maybe you say who cares? You quickly find an excuse, as if they don't like you because you are not rich. Being rich or poor has nothing to do with sexual attraction, but ignorance does.

On the other hand, people in good shape are also very ignorant most of the time. Because of their lack of intelligence, they waste all their temporal physical beauty. When we see someone in good shape, we try to smile because we are attracted. But I'm not saying only a good physique is everything! You could have great humor and personality, which are much better than just a good body shape, in my opinion. But if you had both, wouldn't it be great? In any case, we can discuss personality another day, but now let's focus on our body. Long story short, if you want to have lean muscle you have to watch how much calories you consume a day, a week, and the course of a month, not just how much you exercise! Try to gradually cut down all kind of meat, egg, dairy products, and fish from your daily diet.

CHAPTER II
BORING

♦♦♦

The name of this chapter is maybe a little bit confusing but believe it or not; for most of us, this is a second stage where we can give up. We get bored. Knowing how to deal with this stage is as important as knowing how to exercise and what to eat. As I said, a lifting trophy is a long term goal; it does not happen in a day, week, or month. It takes much longer than that. If you are following a single schedule, you will likely get bored, especially when you don't see many results. The trick is that you need to have fun, you have to enjoy what you are doing, and you need to be in harmony with your body. Thus, you need to understand how it works, not everything is necessary, but whatever is essential to reach the goal. Your body is being programmed to store fat if you have an easy life relaxing all day every day, if you eat and lounge on the sofa, your body will develop soft skin and fat. How do you develop lean muscle, avoid storing fat, and at the same time, not get bored and be in harmony with your body? How do you keep the right balance?

Let's say your dream is to have six-pack abs; your belly is the most challenging part of your body because most of the fat is stored in and around your belly. You can't just do an abs exercise and expect to have a six-pack! You must count your calorie intake and reduce it every day because if you consume more calories than you burn, your body will convert it into fat and store it on top of your abs. We may not see decent abs because of this fat. When I say to reduce calories every day, I mean the reduction of 200-500 calories, not too much. I don't recommend a strict diet to get fast results in short periods. That's because when you are trying to get quick results, you are not in harmony with your body, and it will affect your skin and your face. As soon as you stop dieting, you will regain the weight. Even more, there is an explanation as to why this happens, but I won't go into details because I like to keep it short and straightforward. All you have to do is gradually reduce the calories and try to have fun!

Yes, I mean it exactly as it sounds! Have fun. If you don't feel going to the gym, don't go! If you don't want to eat chicken breast, don't eat it! Try fish instead. Do you want some alcohol? What about a glass of red wine? Try one glass. What about sex? You shouldn't restrict yourself in having sex! Have as much as you like, it will help you to burn calories, sex is an essential component of a healthy lifestyle. It has a lot more benefits, such as reducing stress and heart disease. You will feel happier and healthier. Now, what about a pub beer, some sweet cheesecake, and so on? Well, those things are not great for you, but they're essential for some people to alleviate their boredom and not give up. As a result, that's why we have one red day to eat and drink all of this sugary stuff you love. But you should only do it once a week! In case you can't do without chocolate, try protein bars. Eating one or two protein bars a day is better than eating any other sweets you see on supermarket shelves but don't confuse it for food. There are even food replacement bars. But we should stay away from such a product, companies would do just about anything to make money, but we should be smart not to allow them to do this at the expense of our health. No bars can replace vegetables and a healthy meal.

Today even vegetables and meat are difficult to find because big corporations are investing in making money as quick as possible. So what they do is put animals in cages with minimal space and feed them with genetically modified food to speed up their growth. Vegetables grow in the same way with chemicals. Sometimes they don't even use a field — just shelves in a greenhouse and chemicals. Of course, you can find some organic products to buy if you can afford it. In any case, it's always better to eat fresh organic food, cook if you have time, all you need is half an hour to cook decent food. Please see the green, yellow, and red pages, as to what is right, not so good, and bad for the US. Visualization is as essential as knowing what is right. Knowing what is good for you to eat is one thing but have visualized what is good or bad will have a positive psychological impact. Your memory will remind you every time you go to the market. You will not be easily scammed and misguided with all this marketing bullshit such as green packaging, beautiful, healthy living TV adverts, etc.… How do we measure how much we eat? Of course, we can't use scales every time to determine how much we are eating. There is no time for that, and also, it's annoying. Use measure scoops for oats and nuts, if you are unsure about anything else, use a scale once to weigh the food. For example, let's say you weigh 100g of chicken breast, put it on a plate, and see how 100g of chicken breast would look like on a plate. Visualize it or take a picture of it, so you don't need to use a scale again for next time.

Here is another annoying and ineffective habit. Let's say you eat oatmeal every day, you might be getting bored, but you think it's healthy, maybe you just like it. Eating the same thing every day is not healthy, and there is no fun whatsoever. We need to try and change it up. Let's say oatmeal today and tomorrow Dutch apple pancakes. Doing this is not only fun, but your body will get the nutrition it needs, and it will help you to reduce belly fat.

CHAPTER III
TIME

❖ ❖ ❖

As I said, there are no short cuts, nor healthy short cuts. You can use a diet plan that helps you to lose weight within short periods, but you will regain it even quicker. So we should keep in mind that this is a long term game. I would say lifelong, but I don't want to scare anyone, however, once you get used to it, you will understand what I mean by "lifelong." Starting is difficult, but the rest will be easy and joyful. Living healthy will become your lifestyle. Once you get in shape, you will also be able to eat more freely if you want to. In time, you should master not only nutrition and exercises but the philosophy of a healthy life.

Let's say you are going on an all-inclusive vacation for ten days or so, you book a 5-star hotel with all it has to offer. There are luxury and plenty of food, and unique desserts, lots of varieties and you love all of this, you can eat as much as you like since you already paid for it. At the end of the day, you are on vacation, so you let yourself enjoy and take benefit of everything and of course, you put on some weight. Now you are lazy to run or do any exercise, will you have enough strength to come back and start all over again? As I see, some of my friends did start all over again and some couldn't, they found it too difficult. So there is no guarantee whatsoever of what any of us would do, of what your situation would be like after the vacation. The point I want to make here is that you should not play with your health. You should master the game to know what is a good pleasure and what is a bad pleasure. A bad pleasure is a sugar, no matter what shape it comes in, whether it is chocolate, cake, or whatever. Good pleasures are eating food I have described in green pages, having a calm mind, feeling healthy, wanting to go for a run, and so on. Don't sacrifice your mind and soul for your mouth and belly. Good pleasure is long term happiness! Bad pleasure is short term happiness. To be healthy and be in good shape should be a lifelong choice, not the short-term goal! Lots of people fail because they don't know what they are doing and why they're doing it.

There could be so many reasons why we start going to the gym. Sometimes we see someone that we like, and we want him or her to love us back, assuming that if we're in good shape, they would like us. Sometimes friends or colleagues ask us, "Hey, I'm going to join the gym, would you like to come?" Sure, why not! But then after two months or so they might get fed up and say, "This gym stinks, I should cancel my membership, and I run in the park instead." The park is just an excuse for them to give up. And if you follow them, you are going to do the same thing. There could be many reasons why people fail, but I want to mention some of them in a list. People are jealous when they see that a neighbor has bought a new car. We are often jealous of someone, especially someone we know who has a nicer girlfriend or boyfriend, a good physique. We usually don't care how they obtained the result they have. We want the same thing or better, and as soon as possible. But the matter is that if we're going to succeed, we should change our approach! If someone is in good shape, we shouldn't be jealous.

Instead, we should be inspired. Besides, if someone has muscles, it doesn't mean he is healthy, he could be on steroids. Assuming someone is on steroids is also wrong; in fact, it's not our business how they achieved it. We should do it our way, maybe taking more time, but doing it right. Being healthy is the most important thing. We must do our best to maintain a healthy balance in everything, including food, exercise, work, and sleep, a especially sleep because good quality sleep is an essential part of a healthy lifestyle. Being masculine is only secondary.

CHAPTER IV
STRESS

♦♦♦

We all know that stress is not good for us, but we experience stress from time to time. When we talk about fitness and health, healthy eating and exercising is nothing when it comes to stress. The stress could be a reason that you don't see results. Can stress make you gain weight? Yes, of course. Increased cortisol levels as a result of anxiety cause fat to build up in the stomach. Stress can cause menstrual problems, skin problems such as acne or eczema, depression or anxiety, obesity, diabetes, heart disease, high blood pressure, diarrhea, forgetfulness, frequent aches and pains, headaches, a lack of energy and focus, sexual problems, fatigue, trouble sleeping or sleeping too much, and weight loss or gain. Ok, I got it! It's bad. So what we can do about it? I don't want to be stressed, but I can't control situations, of course, everyone wants to be happy. Life is not easy. You can tell me this and more; there are plenty of excuses like always. Most of them are true if not all. But still, you need to win the trophy; we still need to cross the river. Excuses, blaming the circumstances are things that everyone can do but not you, you are not everyone.

Reading this book makes me think that you are looking for new ways to change your life. The biggest enemy of humanity is to think we know! To think we are better than others, arrogance and greed. By changing your life regarding everything mentioned, you will become human, an intelligent human. Not everyone who speaks and dresses up should be considered human. No, I would call them smart animals, comparing them to an animal species. In terms of wealth, perhaps some animals are richer than humans, that's due to their owners, or fame.

Yes, there are famous animals too, that are TV stars like people. So let me ask you a question: What is the difference between those people who chase after fame and wealth and a dog that is already rich and famous? The dog is already there, but those people have a long way to go! See? By chasing fame, our greed and arrogance would leave us way behind animals. But what if you were to ask questions to yourself as to what is the purpose of your life? Where can I find true happiness? Just by asking questions like this, you would already find yourself way ahead of any famous animals up there.

In my opinion, the purpose of human existence is to find oneself and achieve maximum intelligence. Money, status, and luxury are secondary. If you don't reach your maximum potential, you are neither human nor animal, you will become a soul lost in greed and arrogance, and you will never be fully satisfied with anything no matter how much money, status, or luxury you might have. Stress and anxiety will be with you always, and this will destroy you. On the other hand, if you reach your full potential as an intelligent human, you will become happier. Nobody can upset or stress you. See, your brain determines what is good or bad information and accordingly sends messages through your nervous system. Your mood will change accordingly, as bad info will affect a negative mood and good info will affect a positive mood. There are different ways for information to be created in our mind through reading, watching TV, chatting with people, or thinking yourself an accident. The bad news is easily spread today as everyone is focused on the negative, people find it more exciting, accordingly newspapers and TV channels bombarding us with bad news to have better ratings.

How can we deal with all of the above? The short answer is to not focus your attention on bad! I soon as you detect something is not right, ignore it. Focus only on the good, be the right person. Don't lie, don't do evil to anyone. Let's say someone wronged you and then you pay them back. You probably think that you are not afraid of him or her, you are smarter and stronger, so you pay them back double of what he or she did to you. In this case, what happened is that you let your inner emotions awaken your ego and your ego arouses your nervous system, your brain starts coming up with a plan to destroy the opponent. No matter whether you succeed or not, you are going to lose anyway. If you couldn't manage by destroying him, your ego will not allow you to relax so that more stress will damage your health. In case you succeed, you will be happy just for a short period, that's because the ego is celebrating a win. But it's short-lived because it's not the ego's nature to make you happy. As long as it dominates you, it will find another reason to accuse someone of ignorance or any other fault. Thus trouble starts again and again. We often go to the gym not because we love training but because our ego is in charge because someone you know has a better physique and you want to get the same results. You do this because someone you know is a member of the gym.

When a man is upset, he doesn't care what he eats and drinks, even sleep is difficult for him. When you are angry you might even start smoking, why should you start smoking? Does it help? No, of course not! But the thing is that you can't find your place, you must do something. So, are others smoking? You start, as well. You kind of feel sick and sick men need friends more than ever. Smoking, together with others makes you one step closer to them, not only tobacco but everything you do with others gets you one step closer to them. But it is more likely for you to pick angry and evil people as friends at the time, not peaceful ones. I'm not saying smokers are bad people; smoking is just a bad habit for some people. Breaking things feels good at the time. That's because your ego is in charge of you who has dominion over troubled men enjoys the moment, celebrating the victory. So you feel sick, you destroy and you kind of feel happy. In general, you are not well; physically, there is nothing wrong with you; they're just emotions and the state of your mind. We call it mental breakdown, depression, and anxiety. What is the opposite of this? The opposite of this would be tranquility. Peace of mind! Everything you desire - health, progress in your career or business, a relationship with colleagues, friends, and loved ones - everything will work out just fine if you have peace of mind. So your happiness and accordingly, your success, depending on the state of your mind. Training at the gym, having the best diet plan will not work unless you are in the right state of mind, and the right state of mind is a calm one. Remember that there are ways to improve and have peace of mind, such as meditation, mindfulness and yoga. Here are some short quotes I found interesting that will probably help you improve your wellbeing:

1. You should only count on yourself.
2. If you like someone, tell them.
3. If you miss someone, call them.
4. If you are not sure, ask them to explain.
5. If you want to meet someone, invite them.
6. Do you want something? Ask.
7. Don't argue.
8. What if they don't understand? Explain it to them.
9. Did you make a mistake? Admit it.

10. Remember that everyone has their truth which does not necessarily match yours.
11. Don't be a friend of a fool.
12. The essential things in life are wisdom and love.
13. Your worries are only in your head.
14. Try to enjoy every moment of your life.
15. Remember that you will not have another life.
16. Don't grieve.
17. Remember that you don't owe anything to anyone.
18. Try use time and money to understand the world, universe, kindness, and enjoy it.
19. In life, believe only in yourself.
20. Try to forgive everyone.
21. Live today because yesterday is gone and tomorrow may never come.
22. Remember that today is the best day.

Your brain is not only the organ that needs attention, but it's the most important one because it controls the rest of the organs. It's a door to your soul and universe; if you can control your mind, you can control your sickness and happiness, controlling your mind doesn't imply the calculation of business profits, managing a big company, or successfully accomplishing one particular task! However, there is nothing wrong doing all the above. By controlling your mind, I mean you are fully aware of yourself as one individual, not more or less. You are happy with what you have and don't care about what other people have; you are happy today at the moment. You can breathe, eat, and think. Nothing is impossible if you stay in control of your mind. If you want to have muscles, that's easy, only if you want them for yourself, but if you want them for others, for them to like you, then it's hard. First of all, you will find it difficult to stay in focus in the long term, to exercise regularly, diet, sleep, and so on. And even if you manage to do all this to attract someone, you will not be successful, because if he or she likes you for your good looks, they may not like your personality.

So the best thing is to do whatever you like for yourself, be the best version of yourself. We often say I have to do this now, this is important, once I've finished, that's it, and I will start enjoying myself. I will do all the things I like! Guess what? Once you do whatever you think is important now, something else important will come along and so on. You won't remember what you said months ago, or even if you do, your brain will find another excuse to ignore the promises you made to yourself and will carry on with life, with you always being busy thinking about important things you have to do from day today. Most of the time, we don't acknowledge ourselves as to why we do what we do. Yes, it's not an easy thing to change, because we cannot ignore the things we have done for years and years.

We can't start doing things we had never done before and live a life we have never lived before. But bit by bit we can make changes. Let's say you gave up your job and started looking for another one, something you have never done before, or you have started a business you always wanted. That would be great, but you may find yourself struggling, being stressed at the time, and confused. You will face challenges and make mistakes; it's possible that you will miss the old job that you always hated. It will be stressful that money isn't coming in and you are spending all your savings. You may even decide to go back to your old routine, back to your old job. That's not a problem as long as you don't give up. You have gained experience, maybe feeling defeated, but you haven't given up. You will fight back as soon as you gain energy or acquire the finances you need.

The easiest way is to take steps while you are doing whatever you are doing. Take 10-20% of your earnings and invest in things you are more interested. Are you not sure what it is that you are interested? Or maybe 10-20% is not enough to do what you want to do? In both cases, you can still do something! As you can do something new every day, every day you can go out of your comfort zone! Take a different route to work or home, go to a different coffee shop or restaurant, discover different foods, see a different country, city, or village. Just do something different from what you did yesterday, last week, last month, or last year. This will take you a step closer to finding out what your passion is in case you don't already know yet, or you will gain experience and feel very at ease out of your comfort zone. You will start doing something you enjoy more and more often, not because you have to or for the sake of money, but because this is your passion. This is what you enjoy doing, and this is what makes you feel fulfilled! Doing nothing, rescheduling things for tomorrow, next month, or next year is a loser's game!

Here is one more example of how can you do something new every day and how you can change your habits to something better, to bring pleasure to things you are doing anyway. Most of us like to buy coffee in the morning on the way to a job, some of us like to go to Nero, Starbucks, Costa, and so on. Some will go to McDonald's not because they like it, but because they think it is cheaper! However, they prefer Nero over McDonald's. So how much is cheaper? 50p? Yes, 50p is money, but the coffee you get from McDonald's is not worth any money at all in my opinion, so if you don't have an extra 50p to get better coffee maybe you should consider making it at home by yourself and taking it with you. Anyway, I'm not trying to tell you where to drink your coffee, no! All I'm trying to say is if you want to enjoy a coffee outside then enjoy it, have a quality one with flavor, raise your standards, don't accept something cheap for the sake of money! It's not worth it.

Start meditating. There are plenty of videos, apps, and books that will help you to meditate. Meditation is a powerful tool; it will help you to stand on top of your game. Lots of past toxic information will rise in your mind reminding you of an accident you had, someone who cheated on you, something or someone you have lost, someone who insulted you, and so on. Whenever this kind of information comes to mind, your mood will worsen, and the smile will disappear from your face. Stress levels will increase. You could lose interest in whatever you do, whatever makes you happy, losing a moment, a day, weeks, months, and years. You can't help it, these negative things involuntarily pop into your head and ruin your mood, your life. We should let them go, but we can't. When we overcome with anger we are done, we don't think clearly, we could make stupid mistakes that will cost us years or even our life. So if we start practicing meditation, soon after we will learn how to find peace, how to remain peaceful in challenging situations, and how to be calm. Besides, this is the way to happiness! Sometimes you might hear someone say, yes I want to be angry, I want to destroy him, someone should teach him a lesson, look at what he did! We can go on and on. But the short answer to all this is NO! You don't teach anything to fool, angry men, or a sneaky bastard. No, because you cannot. You will end up disappointed as you can't teach them. Life will! Your game is to be smart and happy, to create value for others and not harm them.

Learn from the experience and mistakes of others.

"Smart people learn from the mistakes of others, average people learn from their mistakes, but fools will never learn."

You can't steal from or deceive people to get rich and be happy at the same time! You become whatever you think all day every day. Whatever you think will happen. So be positive for your own sake.

Let's say you had a car you wanted to sell. It wasn't selling, and one day a very close relative came to you and asked you to sell him the car. He told you that he would make a payment on it every month. You weren't happy about it, thought that he wasn't going to give you back anything and that's exactly what happened. He never gave you any money for the car!

The lesson you could learn from this is that you plaid someone else's game. If you think that you don't trust someone, then stay away from that person no matter who he or she is. If you don't because of your traditions, religion, or whatever, then you are playing someone else's game. Of course, you will lose no matter if it is money, a car, house, or time. Whatever we do, we have to do it willingly and be positive about it. I have a friend who could never say no to people. They used to borrow money from him, and he could never say no, not because he didn't want to but because he was concerned about what would they say about him if he refused. At the end of the day, he had to ask them to return his money. Sometimes some of them did return it, but others never did. You probably have worked somewhere you hate to earn a living, then you have saved some of it as a rainy day fund and now here is someone you know, they could be your old friend, sister, brother, flat mate, and so on. One thing they have in common is that they don't want to do what you are doing and what you have done! They want to have a more comfortable life, to have a business, have a beautiful house, an expensive car, eat well, drink and so on. So to finance their miscalculated lifestyle, they borrow from whomever they can. Don't expect them to care how you earned or saved the money you just gave to them because they won't, unfortunately. So now you have to get it back from them, asking, explaining, begging, fighting, or just giving up. No matter what you do, you have to leave these people as soon as you can, this is the only way! Don't be scared to be alone if you have to, as you were born alone and you will die alone. In the meantime, go to work, do your business, do whatever you have to do to earn a living, live a fulfilling life, and be happy. Read books. Books are your best friends. They can change your life for the better, as they are written by people you have never had the chance to meet. Their life experiences may be better than yours; they might have a better knowledge of having lived in different countries and centuries. The best thing is that you can choose any of those books, unlike friends, as we have mostly chosen them because we studied together or worked together and somehow we think we understand them better than other people. We feel we know these people because we see them more often. However, it doesn't mean that you will always understand them, people change, and so do you.

CHAPTER V
GYM NONSENSE

Are you going to the gym because you want to be healthy and happy? Sure, don't forget to grab some energy drinks that are selling inside of almost every gym. No, not really! Forgive my sarcasm. I mean, how can you sell energy drinks at the gym? A gym is supposed to be a place where we get inspired to live healthily. Instead, on coming in or leaving, we see these stupid poisonous energy drinks and this is just the beginning. They have hundreds of members and one janitor, so everything you touch is stinking. Of course not every gym but most! It's very dangerous to use all the equipment without knowing how to use it. The problem is that most of us think that we know everything. We go there to get the wrong idea of what a healthy life is. We start using protein shakes, creatine, and god knows what, plus we get injured if we are not lucky enough to know how to use sticky machines and dumbbells as there is no one to look after you. Most personal trainers working at a gym are contracted to draw customers to the gym, get more money out of you, and split a commission with the gym, so no one cares what you do or how you do it unless you pay extra for a personal trainer. It's all about the business. Yes, we all understand it's a private enterprise and should have a profit, but maybe they can employ some more people and improve services? Get rid of these poisonous drinks they are selling inside. In any case, I can't tell gym owners how to run their business. But I can tell you that the gym is not the answer. It's not bad if you know what you are doing if it's well looked after, and if it doesn't have a trap contract of a gym membership attached to it. It's like you have bought a new car. When you buy a new car, I understand you have to pay what car is worth, and a percentage on top of it for a bank or whoever finances it for you but paying a fee for a membership at a gym where you cannot go anymore for whatever reason is nothing but a trap! When you want to join, you are tempted to sign better deals, and there is a marketing trick waiting for you. Sign up for 12 months, and you only pay £35 a month or pay £70 a month if you pay as you go. I mean the gym is supposed to be a place for healthiness and happiness, not for extra responsibility and stress. There are healthy alternatives if you have the money to pay a personal trainer. Find them online and meet them at a park, it's better for them and good for you. Or go for a run and do some pushups, there are plenty of exercises you can do in the park. I have seen people coming and going to the gym with no changes to their body whatsoever. That's because they come just for the sake of it, do some treadmill running and some other exercises. Most of the time, they waste time for themselves and others as well, because they sit and occupy the machines. Do you want to tell them to move on? Let me use it if you aren't? Some will tell you they have 1 or 2 more sets to go, and they are still on their cell phone. I don't know about you, but I found it very disappointing as I go to the gym for exercising, not for arguments or fighting. It's annoying.

CHAPTER VI
GO ORGANIC

Somewhere inside in your heart, you know organic is good, but there come false beliefs that organic is not as good as you might think! Organic is expensive! We are bombarded with these sponsored ideas of something artificially grown being almost the same or as good as organic. Or they may even tell you that non-organic is better. As an idea, something grown non-organically being the same or even better, of course, is nonsense, but the problem is that money talks! Non-organically grown products are cheaper, and they're everywhere. It's more profitable and safer for farmers, I mean for people in business and corporations. There are not many honest farmers left; everything has been taken over by the big corporations. Using pesticides is profitable for their business because the product they produce grows faster and has a longer shelf life in warehouses and on shop shelves. It's easy to grow, as it's been designed to grow fast and look beautiful, and no insects can harm vegetables grown on pesticides, so losses are minimal. Of course, they spray lots of human-made chemicals on it, which will end up in our body and blood after a time.

Thus corporations advertise heavily to make you believe that non-organic is as good as organic. We have considerable problems in big cities where we are busy working most of the time. There isn't even enough time to cook for ourselves; all we have left is to grab some ready-made food as long as it smells or tastes good. Who cares what is inside a meal? Even if you do care, there is almost no information on what ingredients did they use to make the hot food. However, there is information on frozen food, but at least fifty percent of us don't understand what half of the ingredients are. Not to mention that along with chemicals and preservatives, there nothing is organic in it. We are talking about food at most of the shops that we consider being healthy and the hot takeaway food which is meant to be healthy. I'm not talking about McDonald's where you can buy a big Mac and fries for two pounds. Anyone in their right mind should know that it's not healthy at all, but yet there is a queue in almost every McDonald's. There is not only McDonald's, but there are also KFC, Burger King, and many more big and small fast-food chains who do everything to make a profit on behalf of our health. That's because they're cheap, they are everywhere, and they have lots of money to spend on advertising. I mean come on, how good can it get by situating well-designed restaurants in the center of such an expensive city as London, and spending as much as two or three pounds for a meal including a drink. But in fact, It's not as cheap as you might think in the long-term considering your health.

Five to ten years down the road, most of us will find ourselves spending much more than we thought we had saved on this unhealthy food. There will be the suffering of pain, both physical and mental when you hear the news that you've been diagnosed with an illness. That could be anything, even cancer, which could lead to death! Some of my readers may think that I'm overly dramatic, that if it's so dangerous, why does the government allow it? In my opinion, there are many different factors as to why the government cannot do much, even if they want to. When it comes to eating and drinking, we can't solely rely on the government or anybody else. We need to educate ourselves. Either we rely on the government if it's approved and legally sold or we adapt to twenty-first-century reality. The changes were made long ago, unfortunately, and now things are not as simple as they seem. We can't just blame one government or form a new one to ban non-organic and fast food chains. Can you imagine what would happen if one day your government decides to get rid of these fast junk food chains? Hundreds of thousands of people would be in the streets without a job. Who is going to pay their mortgage? And then who is going to supply healthy organic food? There is not enough right now. We now just realize that all this pollution and plastic waste is destroying our planet. Governments all around the world are trying to tackle this issue, but it will take time. In the meanwhile, many animals will die, including birds and fish. Humans are supposed to be the most intelligent species on this planet, but we are the ones who are destroying the world and ourselves.

As I said above, we need to educate ourselves! The more educated we are, the more we will demand organic products. When demand rises, supply will follow. Businesses will adapt. No one has to lose a job or stay hungry. To make it clear once again, try to buy organic! Increase the demand and change your future and the future of next generation. When McDonald's or any other corporation see a market for an organically produced product is growing, and their businesses start to decline, they will change the menu, they will invest in organic. Don't ask politicians to do much, they cannot and won't do it. We don't want to hear more lies; it's a waste of time. How did we get here, and where are we? By poisoning and destroying the planet! Three huge problems - the love of power, greed, and ignorance - got us to where we are right now. Most of our politicians love power. The people who have most of the money are greedy. These people and politicians work together. Money lovers need favorable rules to make a hundred percent of profits, to package a poison as the healthiest food, and make millions and billions at the expense of our health. On the other hand, politicians need donors to run their political campaigns, so they become ignorant for the sake of power. Both money and political power go hand in hand, passing on to the generations. That's why we are here in this situation. Do you know why they are trying to tackle climate change now? Because they have just realized that we are all going to die, it's as simple as that. Including them! New planets similar to earth are not in reach of humans for them to escape, so they have no choice other than to fix what we have destroyed right here on earth. Anyway, are these politicians and people in business all so cruel? What about new entrepreneurs who do business or work a job because of their passion for a product or a country they love and not for the sake of money? Well, yes, there are people like this, but they are a minority, like us, organic eaters. Those politicians will not have enough power and support to make significant changes, and big sharks will replace them in the coming elections. Do you think that we are choosing our representatives in Parliament? No, we are not. Money does. And who has money? Big corporations. The same goes for enterprises. They are okay as long as they remain small. When they grow, investors come on board, and the game changes. Even if founders don't destroy each other and get greedy, they will be left with a minimum percentage and not be able to do much. Most of the time, people like this would walk away from their invention or be pushed out. The best scenario is to remain small.

Now, let's start a new revolution, and this time we shall demand organic. Of course, we don't need to go into the streets and start throwing stones. Instead, next time we go shopping, we should try to find what organic products they do have. If you have no luck finding anything, most likely that's because they don't have it, but still, try and ask the shop assistant for help. The more we ask, the more they will realize that customers are getting smarter, that customers are looking for organic. So shop managers will have no choice but to include customer inquiries in their reports to senior management. Once the message passes through management to suppliers and investors, they will demand current suppliers and farmers to change the way they cultivate and supply organic products. The changes are not going to happen tomorrow; it will take time. But the point is that it will happen. As demand increases, supply will follow.

All we have to do is to buy one thing, let's say one pack of organic carrots or ask what organic products they have in stock. The last time I went to three supermarket chains in central London, I found only one organic product, and it was a pack of carrots. Just forty pence were more expensive than nonorganic carrots. I had no choice but to buy one package of organic carrots with the other vegetables being nonorganic as I didn't have a choice. At this time, when we have no choice but to buy all non-organic, what can one pack of organic carrots do for you? In my opinion, it can do a lot not just for you but for the farmer behind these carrots and for the next generation. It is not only super healthy for you, but the farmer who sells organically grown products will be encouraged to grow a larger variety of products. Which means next year you could find another variety of organic vegetables in the store, and in time your kids could have plenty of choices to eat healthily.

CHAPTER VII
GREEN PAGES

The green, yellow, and red pages are just an illustration as to what is good, not so good, and wrong for us. Of course, this is not a full list of all foods. You are welcome to do your research on any food that is not on this list and find something else that is healthy so you can include it in your menu. The goal of making this list is to make people think about healthy options in terms of the food. This may not be a full list, but it will be enough to choose from and include in your daily menu, to start living healthy. Form your own opinion as to what is good for you and don't pay much attention to what each shop consultant wants to tell you. Each shop is full of processed, packaged, and preserved food, as this is the way to create value for a business, to keep food for long periods on the shelves, for months and even years. Modern science has made it possible to extract or add vitamins. However, this is not entirely bad! This would be good for military rations, traveling, or hiking for some time, but eating all this junk all day every day as a regular routine is a severe mistake. It is a lack of education, ignorance, and laziness to cook. In any big or small store, you will see a tiny part of the shop shelves taken up by food in the green and yellow categories. Even if it looks like green, it's not organic, because most of these products are just rapidly grown, these are unnatural vegetables and fruits that last a long time on shelves. The same goes for meat and milk products. So my question is that if we are being cheated on the so-called live, green food, that it's supposed to be natural and healthy, what are we eating when we buy processed packaged food such as ready-to-eat food, protein and chocolate bars, any cookies, conserved fish, meat, cheese, or you name it? My easy guess is that it isn't healthy at all. Half of the ingredients written on the back of it are not even understandable for most of us as to what these things are and how healthy they are for the human body. There are things we don't know, such as the conditions in which this food product was processed and what healthy ingredients have been used. The damage might cause you are unknown.

I used to work in a sandwich factory in London where our factory supplied leading supermarket chains in London. Guess what? Since I saw what went on there, I have never repurchased a sandwich in a shop. We use to have gloves, let's say there are five people on the line depending on the sandwich, there could be more people. One person puts on one ingredient, like cheese, and the line runs quite fast. I saw people run into the bathroom and come back without washing their hands because they were running out of time and being lazy. When I asked why they didn't wash, the excuse was that they didn't have the time. Or they would say, "What is the problem? They use gloves anyway." But before you put gloves on your hands you touch them with your dirty hands, don't you? Some of them even ate sandwich ingredients from the boxes in the fridge, and so on. But they had another problem, they were tired of standing on their feet in the refrigerator, workers didn't get much of a break, and they hated the job they were doing. They weren't going to buy those sandwiches anyway, why would they care.

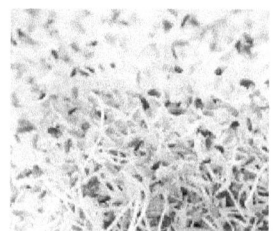 **Alfalfa.**

Alfalfa is usually consumed by people as a natural supplement or in the form of alfalfa sprouts. They are generally high in vitamin K and additionally include many different nutrients, including vitamin C, copper, manganese, and folate. Thiamin, riboflavin, magnesium and iron.

Alfalfa also has an excessive content material of bioactive plant compounds. They include saponins, coumarins, flavonoids, phytosterols, phytoestrogens, and alkaloids. Alfalfa May Help Lower Cholesterol, Improve Metabolic Health, and Relive Menopause Symptoms.

However, you should avoid Alfalfa if you are pregnant due to the fact it may cause uterine stimulation or contractions. Therefore, it should be avoided in the course of pregnancy.

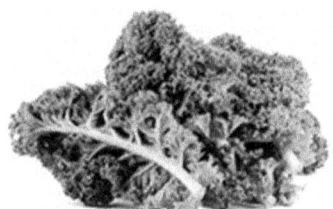 **Kale**

Kale Is a best sources of vitamin K. Loaded with powerful antioxidants such as Quercetin and kaempferol. Vitamin C. Kale can help lower cholesterol; May reduce the risk of heart disease.

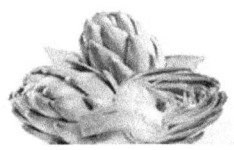 **Artichokes.**

Artichokes are nutritionally dense, composed of various vitamins and minerals. They are a good source of Vitamin B6, calcium, and iron.

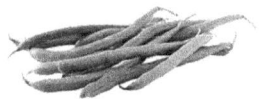 **Green beans.**

Green beans contain many necessary vitamins, which includes folate. One cup of uncooked green beans consists of 33 micrograms of folate, almost ten percent of day by day endorsed value. Folate is a B vitamin that helps stop neural tube defects and other birth defects. One cup of raw green beans gives 690 IU of Vitamin A. vitamin K: 43 mcg.

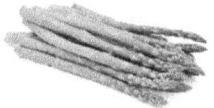 **Asparagus.**

Asparagus is packed full of goodness consisting of vitamin A, an essential nutrient that helps to defend our eyes, skin and immune system, plus vitamin C which helps to support our capillaries and is involved in collagen formation. Asparagus is additionally a desirable supply of vitamin K, used in bone formation and blood clotting.

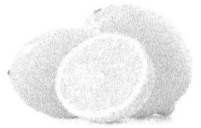

Lemons.

Lemons are a good source of vitamin C and of flavonoids and antioxidants, which are thought to enhance health and wellness in countless ways.

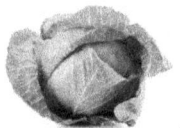

Cabbage.

Cabbage is a top source of manganese, dietary fiber, calcium, magnesium, and potassium. It is additionally rich in a range of vitamins together with vitamin C, B6, A, K, and E. With a 100gram serving of cabbage containing about 25 calories. It is additionally high in antioxidants together with flavonoid, zeaxanthin, lutein, choline, and beta-carotene.

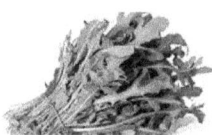

Arugula.

Arugula is rich with vitamin K content. Vitamin K is intimately concerned in calcium regulation and metabolism and helps get the mineral into your bones and preserve it there. Low vitamin K consumption can lead to crippling osteoporosis later in life and is implicated in many different degenerative diseases.

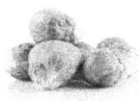

Brussels sprouts.

Brussels sprouts are mainly high in protein when in contrast to different green vegetables. There is a range of health benefits associated with Brussels sprouts, which includes eye and bone protection.

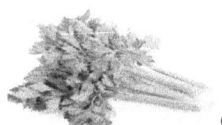

Celery.

Celery is a rich source of phenolic phytonutrients that have antioxidant and anti-inflammatory properties. These phytonutrients include caffeic acid, cinnamic acid, apigenin, luteolin, quercetin, kaempferol, beta-sitosterol and furanocoumarins. Celery is a good source of vitamin K and molybdenum, folate, potassium, dietary fiber, manganese, and pantothenic acid. Celery is also a good source of vitamin B2, copper, vitamin C, vitamin B6, calcium, phosphorus, magnesium, and vitamin A.

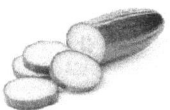

Cucumber.

Cucumber health benefits include decreasing the chance of cardiovascular disease, healthful weight management, detoxifying the body, enhancing the skin, helping eye health, alkalizing the blood, and treating cancer. Other benefits consist of combating horrific breath, aiding digestion, controlling blood sugar level, aiding bones, repairing hair, nails, and dental health.

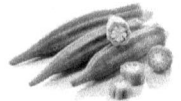 **Okra.**

The health benefits of okra include its ability to improve digestive health and vision, control diabetes, refine pores and skin health, soothe joint pain, stop certain cancers, and make stronger bones. Additionally improves cardiovascular health, balances cholesterol levels, aids the immune system, lowers blood pressure, and protects heart health.

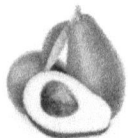 **Avocado.**

The pinnacle health benefits of avocado include its ability to enhance heart health, improve digestion, prevent cancer, enhance liver health, and assist in weight management. Avocado also helps maintain the eyes healthy; due to its excessive lutein content protects the pores and skin from signs of aging. It is a rich source of appropriate fats, vitamins, minerals, antioxidants, and Phytol sterols.

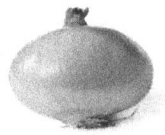

Onion.

The stunning health benefits of onions consist of their ability to treat and prevent cancer, heart disorders, and diabetes. They additionally deal with the frequent cold, asthma, bacterial infections, respiratory problems, angina, and cough.

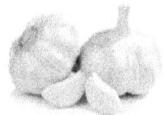

Garlic.

Alien, in garlic, offers innumerable health benefits which include combating cold and cough, reducing blood pressure, conflict coronary heart ailments, and stopping Alzheimer's. It also helps relieve earaches, treat intestinal issues, cure wounds, prevent cancer, and reduce excess gas.

Banana.

Health benefits of banana include assisting with weight loss, decreasing obesity, curing intestinal disorders, relieving constipation, and curing prerequisites like dysentery, anemia, tuberculosis, arthritis, gout, and kidney and urinary disorders. Banana can additionally help with menstrual troubles and burns. It is suitable for reducing blood pressure, protecting coronary heart health, boosting metabolism and immunity, lowering the severity of ulcers, ensuring healthy eyes, constructing sturdy bones, and detoxifying the body.

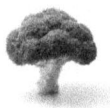

Broccoli.

Broccoli is noticeably rich in dietary fiber and proteins like tryptophan. According to the USDA national nutrient database, it also consists of vitamin A, beta-carotene, lutein zeaxanthin, thiamine, riboflavin, niacin, and pantothenic acid. Along with that, it includes vitamin B6, folate vitamin B9, vitamin C, vitamin E, vitamin B1, and vitamin K. Minerals in it include calcium, iron, magnesium, zinc, sodium, potassium, and phosphorus. It additionally comprises healthy omega-3 fatty acids.

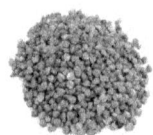

Buckwheat.

Buckwheat is a very nutrient-rich, gluten-free plant with major health benefits, including heart health, reduction of blood pressure, weight loss, prevention of certain cancers and diabetes. Improves digestion and cholesterol levels, aids stronger immune system. Its great range of proteins, minerals, and antioxidants assist in pores and skin and hair health, removing of gallstones, protection from allergies attacks, and remedy from constipation and different intestinal conditions.

Buckwheat is a very desirable source of manganese and copper, magnesium and phosphorus. The buckwheat is loaded with high-quality protein, containing all eight fundamental amino acids, which include lysine.

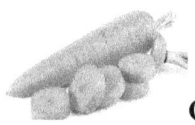 **Carrots.**

Raw carrots are high in vitamin A, which supports health of your eyes and helps the growth of cells. Carrots are low in calories and good source of potassium, magnesium, vitamins C, E, and K. Potassium helps stability the quantities of sodium and water in your blood, which helps modify blood pressure. Magnesium supports healthy bones and coronary heart, essential to muscle function. Vitamins C and E are powerful antioxidants which preserve your cells clear of free radicals and assist slow the symptoms of aging. In addition, raw carrot provides fiber, which helps you feel full, slows down the absorption of sugars.

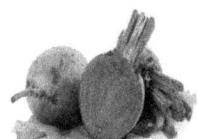 **Beet Roots.**

Beetroots comprise valuable vitamins that may help lower your blood pressure, combat cancer and inflammation, raise your stamina, and help detoxification. Beet veggies are equally, if not more nutritious with vitamins that may also fortify your immune system, aid brain, and bone health.

Beetroots have the highest sugar content material of all vegetables, so they should be eaten in moderation.

Try including beetroots raw to salads or as a phase of your vegetable juice; beet veggies can be mixed with spinach or Swiss chard.

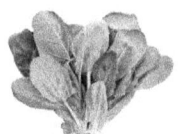 **Spinach.**

Spinach health benefits include aiding detoxification, supporting weight loss, keeping the eye healthy, supporting strong bones, reducing hypertension, promoting good sleep, boosting immunity, promoting youthful health, combating hair loss, curing acne, and enhancing the skin.

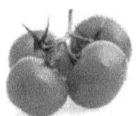 **Tomatoes.**

Tomatoes are a gorgeous natural source of vitamins A, C, and K. Additionally; tomatoes have a lot of folates, potassium, Omega 6 fatty acids, fiber, and manganese. Plus, they are high in water content, low in calories, and have no cholesterol.

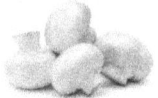 **Mushrooms.**

Mushrooms are the leading source of the antioxidant selenium. Antioxidants, like selenium protects body cells from harm that may lead to continual illnesses and help to strengthen the immune system, as well. In addition, mushrooms grant ergothioneine naturally occurring antioxidant that may also help defend the body's cells.

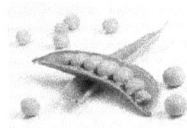

Green Peas.

Green peas are clearly an important phytonutrient source. Flavanols (including catechin and epicatechin), phenolic acids (including caffeic and ferulic acid), and carotenoids (including alpha- and beta-carotene) are among the phytonutrients provided by green peas. Even more unique to this food are its saponins, Pisum saponins I and II. The polyphenol coumestrol is also provided in enormous amounts of this phytonutrient-rich food.

Green peas are an excellent supply of vitamin K, manganese, dietary fiber, vitamin B1, copper, vitamin C, phosphorus, and folate. They are also the good source of vitamin B6, niacin, vitamin B2, molybdenum, zinc, protein, magnesium, iron, potassium, and choline.

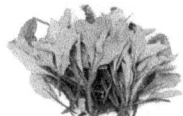

Beet Greens.

Beet vegetables are an incredible source of vitamin K, vitamin A, vitamin C, copper, potassium, manganese, vitamin B2, magnesium, vitamin E, fiber and calcium. They are a very suitable source of iron, vitamins B1, B6, and pantothenic acid, as well as phosphorus and protein. Beet veggies are also a good source of zinc, folate and vitamin B3.

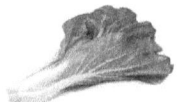

Bok Choy.

Bok Choy is a superb source of Vitamin C, A and manganese, and an excellent source of zinc. Bok choy provides us core different phytonutrient antioxidants.

It's a source of vitamin K, potassium, folate, vitamin B6, calcium and manganese. Iron, vitamin B2, phosphorus, fiber, and protein as well as of choline, magnesium, niacin, vitamin B1, copper, omega-3 fatty acids, zinc, and pantothenic acid. Bok choy also offers flavonoids together with quercetin, kaempferol, and isorhamnetin, and numerous antioxidant phenolic acids, which includes hydroxycinnamic and malic acid.

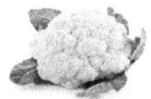

Cauliflower.

The phytonutrients provided through cauliflower are headed off via its glucosinolates. These sulfur-containing compounds are properly studied and known to supply a range of health benefits. Cauliflower is an extremely good source of vitamin C, vitamin K, folate, pantothenic acid, and vitamin B6. It is a very suitable source of choline, dietary fiber, omega-3 fatty acids, manganese, phosphorus, and biotin. Additionally, it is the good source of vitamin B1, B2, and B3, the minerals potassium and magnesium, and protein.

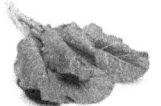

Collard greens.

Based on a very small variety of research looking especially at collard greens, and a large range of studies looking at cruciferous greens as a group, collard greens supply exclusive nutrients that supports for three systems that are closely linked with most cancer prevention. These three structures are one the body's detox system, two its antioxidant system, and three anti-inflammatory systems. Among all sorts of cancer, prevention of the following most cancer types are most carefully related with consumption of collard greens: bladder cancer, breast cancer, colon cancer, lung cancer, prostate cancer, and ovarian cancer.

Collard vegetables are an extremely good source of vitamin K, vitamin A (in the form of carotenoids), manganese, vitamin C, dietary fiber, and calcium. In addition, collard greens are an excellent source of vitamin B1, vitamin B6, and iron. They are good source of vitamin E, copper, protein, magnesium, phosphorus, vitamin B5, folate, omega-3 fatty acids, niacin, vitamin B1, and potassium. Phytonutrients in collard veggies include phenols like caffeic and ferulic acid, flavonoids like quercetin and kaempferol, and glucosinolates like glucobrassicin and glucoraphanin.

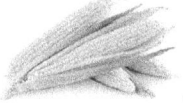

Corn.

Antioxidant phytonutrients are provided through all varieties of corn. The actual phytonutrient combination, however, relies upon on the variety itself. Yellow corn is richer in carotenoids, especially lutein and zeaxanthin. Blue corn has special concentrations of anthocyanins, mainly cyanidin-3-glucosides. Other phytonutrients normally found in corn include organic acids like ferulic, and coumaric acid, and the flavonoid quercetin. Corn is the good source of pantothenic acid, phosphorus, niacin, dietary fiber, manganese, and vitamin B6.

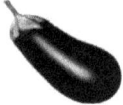
Eggplant.

In addition to the nutrition and minerals, eggplant also contains vital phytonutrients, many of which have antioxidant activity. Phytonutrients contained in eggplant encompass phenolic compounds, such as caffeic and chlorogenic acid.

Eggplant is good source of dietary fiber, vitamin B1, and copper. It is a desirable source of manganese, vitamin B6, niacin, potassium, folate, and vitamin K.

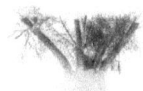
Fennel.

Fennel is a super source of vitamin C. It is also a very good of dietary fiber, potassium, molybdenum, manganese, copper, phosphorus, and folate. In addition, fennel is a good source of calcium, pantothenic acid, magnesium, iron, and niacin.

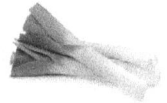
Leeks.

Leeks contain an amazing quantity of polyphenols, together with the flavonoid kaempferol. The widespread amount of sulfur found in leeks can also play an important role in assist of our body's antioxidant and detox structures as well as the formation of our connective tissue. Leeks are an exquisite source of vitamin K. They are good source of manganese, vitamin B6, C, copper, iron, and folate, vitamin A, carotenoids, dietary fiber, magnesium, vitamin E, calcium, and omega-3 fatty acids.

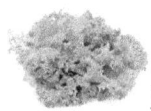

Mustard Greens.

Mustard greens are a superb supply of many vitamins along with vitamin A, K, C and E. They are also an outstanding source of the minerals copper, manganese and calcium. They are a very desirable source of dietary fiber, phosphorus, vitamin B1, B6, and B2. Iron as well as a desirable supply of potassium, magnesium, niacin, pantothenic acid, and folate. In the phytonutrient category, mustard veggies are a valuable source of glucosinolates, which includes sinigrin, gluconasturtiin, and glucotropaeolin. They additionally supply the phenolic acids caffeic and ferulic acid, as well as the flavonoids isorhamnetin, quercetin, and kaempferol.

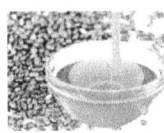

Chia Seed oil.

Cold-pressed organic Chia seed oil carries quintessential fatty acids omega-3 and omega-6, as well as antioxidants known as tocopherols; In fact, it has the highest ranges of antioxidants in the oil family. Chia oil is good for pores and skin hydration, it minimizes trans-epidermal water loss and increases skin barrier function, it strengthens your skin. Omega-3 is an anti-aging property and anti-inflammatory. Chia oil is a good source of treatment for irritated and inflamed skin.

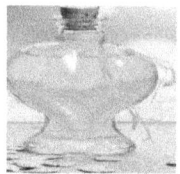
Pumpkin Seed oil.

Pumpkin seed oil includes lowering cholesterol, easing symptoms of benign prostatic hyperplasia (BPH) in men, lowering hot flashes and hormone-related complications in women, and reversing hair loss. The pumpkin seed oil contains phytosterols, which are structurally similar to the body's cholesterol. Phytosterols compete with cholesterol for absorption in the digestive system, which can block cholesterol absorption and lower cholesterol levels. Relief of menopausal symptoms, urinary tract health, possible treatment for metabolic disease, possible treatment for blood pressure, prevention of heart disease. Pumpkin seed oil contains a lot of antioxidants, a decent amount of polyunsaturated fatty acids, potassium, vitamin B2, and folate.

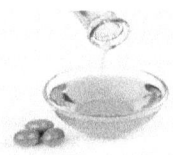
Extra virgin olive oil.

Among the large listing of phytonutrients provided to us by using more virgin olive oil (EVOO), no classes of nutrients are extra essential than its phenols and polyphenols. Most of these phenols and polyphenols supply us with anti-inflammatory benefits, mainly related to reduce irritation in our cardiovascular system. Many of these anti-inflammatory phenols and polyphenols have been the subject of heating research and have discovered to be broken in large quantities with the heating of EVOO. It's good to avoid cooking with EVOO.

Olive oil is also special plant oil in terms of its fat composition, containing about three-fourths of its fats in the form of oleic acid (a monounsaturated, omega-9 fat). It is also a desirable source of vitamin E.

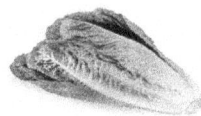 **Romaine lettuce.**

Want to maximize the health advantages of your salads? Start with romaine lettuce because it's packed with nutrients.

Due to its extremely low-calorie content material and high water volume, romaine lettuce—while frequently disregarded in the nutrition world—is genuinely a very nutritious food. Based on its nutrient richness, it's a brilliant source of vitamin A, vitamin K, folate, and molybdenum. Romaine lettuce is additionally a very suitable source of dietary fiber, minerals (manganese, potassium, copper, and iron), and three nutritional vitamins biotin, vitamin B1, and vitamin C.

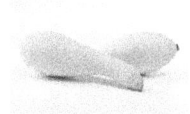 **Summer squash.**

In terms of nutrient richness, some people would no longer place summer squash on their listing of attention-grabbing vegetables. Much greater probable to be protected in this list would be veggies like kale or spinach or broccoli. However, summer squash is a vegetable with extraordinary nutrient richness. Summer squash is an outstanding source of two minerals (copper and manganese) and very suitable or accurate supply of six extra minerals: magnesium, phosphorus, potassium, zinc, calcium, and iron.

In the nutrition category, it's important to see the range of B-vitamins provided with the aid of summer squash. These B-vitamins are B1, B2, B3, B6, pantothenic acid, choline, and folate. (The solely unranked B-vitamins for summer squash are B12 and biotin.) Other vitamins include C and K.

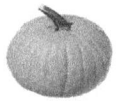

Winter squash.

In the vitamin category, B vitamins are a winter squash specialty. Here we are speaking about the position of winter squash as a very suitable source of vitamin B6, B2, B3, folate, and pantothenic acid. Also, it's necessary to mention in this diet category is vitamin C, which winter squash provides in a very suitable amount; and vitamin A, which winter squash presents in an amazing amount due to its rich array of carotenoids. Vitamin K is also an excellent quantity in winter squash.

One final piece of statistics in this nutrition category for winter squash includes its vitamin E content. While more substantial quantities of vitamin E are provided by way of the seeds of this vegetable.

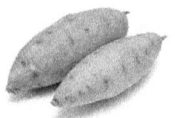

Sweet potatoes.

Sweet potatoes supply some surprising health benefits: antioxidants, anti-inflammatory nutrients, and blood sugar-regulating nutrients.

The orange-flesh of sweet potatoes are extraordinarily prosperous in beta-carotene. The purple-flesh types are awesome sources of anthocyanins, particularly peonidin and cyanidin. Both sorts of sweet potatoes are rich in unique phytonutrients, which include polysaccharide-related molecules referred to as batatins. Sweet potatoes also consist of storage proteins referred to as sporamins that have unique antioxidant properties. Sweet potatoes are a good source of vitamin A. They are also a very desirable source of vitamin C, manganese, copper, pantothenic acid, and vitamin B6. Additionally, they are a good supply of potassium, dietary fiber, niacin, vitamin B1, vitamin B2, and phosphorus.

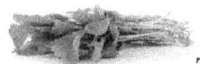

Turnip Greens.

The turnip greens are a great supply of vitamin K, vitamin A (in the form of beta-carotene), vitamin C, folate, copper, manganese, dietary fiber, calcium, vitamin E and vitamin B6. They are a very excellent source of potassium, magnesium, pantothenic acid, vitamin B2, iron, phosphorus: B1, omega-3 fatty acids, niacin, and protein.

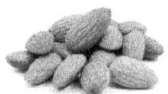

Almonds.

Almonds are high in monounsaturated fats, the identical kind of health-promoting fat as are discovered in olive oil, which has been associated with decreased threat of heart disease. Five large human epidemiological studies, consisting of the Nurses' health study, the Iowa health study, the Adventist health study, and the Physicians health study, all discovered that nut consumption is linked to decrease danger for heart disease. Doctors who studied records estimated that substituting nuts for an equivalent quantity of carbohydrate in a common diet resulted in a 30% reduction in heart ailment risk. Researchers calculated even greater outstanding threat reduction of 45% when fat from nuts used to be substituted for saturated fats (found mainly in meat and dairy products).

Almonds are a very suitable source of vitamin E, manganese, biotin, and copper. Almonds are a suitable supply of magnesium, molybdenum, riboflavin (vitamin B2), and phosphorus. Although a one-quarter cup of almonds includes about 11 grams of heart-healthy monounsaturated fat.

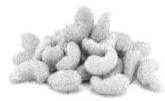 **Cashews.**

Approximately 82% of cashew fats are unsaturated fatty acids, plus about 66% of these unsaturated fatty acids are heart-healthy monounsaturated fats. Monounsaturated fat is good when introducing to a low-fat diet, it can assist in limiting high triglyceride levels. As we know triglycerides are a form, in which fats are carried in the blood, and excessive triglyceride stages are related with a multiplied chance for heart disease, so ensuring you have some monounsaturated fat in your food plan by means of enjoying cashews is an excellent idea, especially for individuals with diabetes.

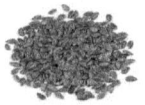 **Flaxseeds.**

Among frequently eaten foods, flaxseeds are an unparalleled source of fiber-related polyphenols called lignans. They are additionally an uncommon supply of mucilaginous gums like arabinoxylans.

Flaxseeds are a great source of omega-3 necessary fatty acids. They are a very desirable supply of dietary fiber, vitamin B1, and copper. They are also a right source of the minerals magnesium, phosphorus, and selenium.

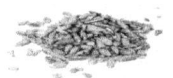

Sunflower Seeds.

Sunflower seeds are a good source of vitamin E and a very suitable source of copper and vitamin B1. In addition, sunflower seeds are an appropriate source of manganese, selenium, phosphorus, magnesium, vitamin B6, folate, and niacin.

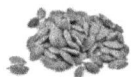

Pumpkin Seeds.

The pumpkin seeds comprise a good variety of antioxidant phytonutrients, inclusive of the phenolic acids hydroxybenzoic, caffeic, coumaric, ferulic, sinapic, protocatechuic, vanillic and syringic acid; and the lignans pinoresinol, lariciresinol. Pumpkins seeds additionally comprise health-supportive phytosterols, which include beta-sitosterol, sitostanol, and avenasterol. Pumpkin seeds are very excellent source of phosphorus, magnesium, manganese, and copper. They are additionally a suitable source of other minerals together with zinc and iron. In addition, pumpkin seeds are an excellent source of protein.

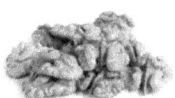

Walnuts.

Walnuts are a notable source of anti-inflammatory omega-3 critical fatty acids, in the shape of alpha-linolenic acid (ALA). Walnuts are also rich in antioxidants, together with being a very suitable source of manganese and copper. They are additionally an excellent source of molybdenum and the B vitamin biotin. Many other minerals are provided by using walnuts in precious amounts. These minerals consist of calcium, chromium, iron, magnesium, phosphorus, potassium, selenium, vanadium, and zinc. In terms of phytonutrients, walnuts contain antioxidant and anti-inflammatory compounds, inclusive of more than a dozen phenolic acids, numerous tannins especially ellagitannins, a large range of flavonoids and vitamin E.

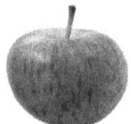 **Apple.**

Apple polyphenols are standout vitamins in this extensively cherished fruit. These polyphenols plus flavonols and especially quercetin of course. Also kaempferol and myricetin), catechins (especially epicatechin), anthocyanins (if the apples are red-skinned), chlorogenic acid, phloridzin, and quite a few dozen extra health-supportive polyphenol nutrients. Apple is an excellent source of fiber, together with both soluble and insoluble pectins, and it's also an excellent source of vitamin C. Apple vitamins are disproportionately present in the skin, which is an especially valuable phase of the fruit with admire to its nutrient content.

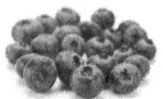 **Blueberries.**

Blueberries provide us with a super variety of phytonutrients, which includes stilbenoids like pterostilbene and flavonoids like quercetin, myricetin, and kaempferol. I would like to clarify that Blueberry anthocyanins are among the most unique of these phytonutrients, and they include cyanidin, malvidin, delphinidin, pelargonidin, peonidin, and petunidin. Blueberries are a very desirable source of vitamin K, vitamin C, and manganese as well as a desirable source of fiber and copper.

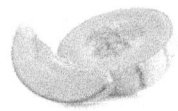

Cantaloupe.

Cantaloupe carries an extensive variety of antioxidant and anti-inflammatory phytonutrients, consisting of the carotenoids alpha-carotene, beta-carotene, lutein, beta-cryptoxanthin and zeaxanthin; the flavonoid luteolin; the organic acids ferulic and caffeic acid; and two cucurbitacins—cucurbitacin B and cucurbitacin E. Cantaloupe is a magnificent source of vitamin A (in the shape of carotenoids) and vitamin C. It is also a good source of potassium, dietary fiber, vitamin B1, vitamin B3 (niacin), vitamin B6, folate, magnesium, copper and vitamin K.

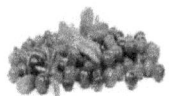

Cranberry.

Cranberry offers us with a brilliant array of phytonutrients. Cranberries are a very suitable source of vitamin C, dietary fiber, and manganese, an excellent source of vitamin E, vitamin K, copper, and pantothenic acid.

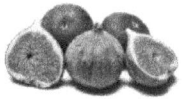

Figs.

The Figs are a good source of dietary fiber, vitamin B6, including copper, potassium, manganese and pantothenic acid.

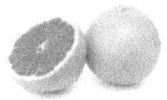

Grapefruit.

Grapefruit is a notable source of vitamin A and vitamin C. It is additionally an excellent source of pantothenic acid, copper, dietary fiber, potassium, biotin and vitamin B1. Grapefruit additionally includes phytochemicals which include limonoids and lycopene.

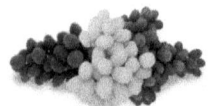

Grapes.

Grapes are an incredible source of phytonutrients, particularly phenols and polyphenols. What are the five basic phytonutrient groups that grapes offer? These are flavanols, flavonoids, phenolic acids, stilbenes, and carotenoids. Grape flavonoids include catechins, epicatechins, procyanidins, quercetin, and petunidin. Grape phenolic acids include coumaric acid, caffeic acid, ferulic acid, and gallic acid. Stilbenes in grapes consist of resveratrol, piceatannol, and pterostilbene. The carotenoids beta-carotene, lutein, and zeaxanthin are also provided in precious amounts in many types of grapes. Grapes are a very desirable source of vitamin K and copper as well as a good source of vitamin B2.

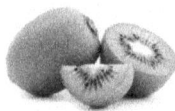

Kiwifruit.

Kiwifruit is a fantastic supply of vitamin C and vitamin K as well as a very desirable source of copper and dietary fiber. Vitamin E, potassium, folate, and manganese.

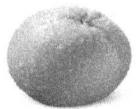
Oranges.

Oranges are a magnificent source of Vitamin C. They are also a very suitable supply of dietary fiber. In addition, oranges are a desirable supply of vitamin B1, pantothenic acid and folate as well as vitamin A, calcium, copper, and potassium.

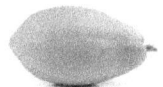
Papaya.

Papaya is a wonderful source of vitamin A (in the structure of carotenoids) and vitamin C. It is a very desirable source of folate. In addition, it is a desirable source of dietary fiber, magnesium, potassium, copper, and vitamin K.

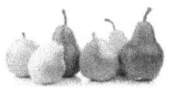
Pears.

The pears are a concentrated supply of phenolic phytonutrients, consisting of hydroxybenzoic acids chlorogenic acid, gentisic acid, syringic acid, and vanillic acid. Carotenoids, beta-carotene, lutein, zeaxanthin. Pears are a very desirable source of dietary fiber and a top source of copper, vitamin C, and vitamin K.

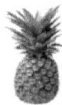

Pineapple.

The pineapple is a great source of vitamin C and manganese. It is additionally a very suitable source of copper and a desirable supply of vitamin B1, vitamin B6, dietary fiber, folate, and pantothenic acid.

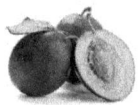

Plums.

Plums are a very excellent source of vitamin C. They are also an excellent supply of vitamin K, copper, dietary fiber, and potassium.

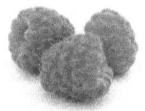

Raspberries.

Raspberries are an amazing source of phytonutrients, with dozens of anthocyanins, flavonoids, stilbenoids, (phenolic acids, tannins, and lignans. They are a surprisingly concentrated supply of ellagitannins (like ellagic acid), cyanidin and pelargonidin. Raspberries are an extremely good source of vitamin C, manganese, and dietary fiber. They are a very desirable source of copper and vitamin K, pantothenic acid, biotin, vitamin E, magnesium, folate, and omega-3 fatty acids.

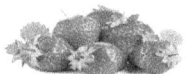

Strawberries.

Strawberries supply us with a rich range of phytonutrients, which includes dozens of polyphenolic antioxidants belonging to the following nutrient groups: flavonoids, phenolic acids, lignans, tannins, and stilbenes. Strawberries are a first-rate source of vitamin C an awesome source of manganese; a very desirable supply of fiber, iodine, and folate; and a suitable supply of copper, potassium, biotin, phosphorus, magnesium, vitamin B6, and omega-3 fats.

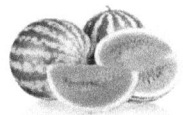

Watermelon.

Watermelon is fruit that is a very good source of the carotenoid lycopene and a rich source of phenolic antioxidants. It contains amino acid citrulline, vitamin C, pantothenic acid, copper, biotin, potassium, vitamin A, vitamin B1, vitamin B6, and magnesium.

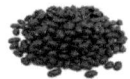

Black Beans.

Among all groups of food often eaten worldwide, no group has a more health-supportive protein and fiber then black beans. Serving a single cup of black beans, you get almost 15 grams of fiber and over 15 grams of protein.

 **Lentils.**

Lentils are a small however nutritionally mighty member of the legume family, they are very desirable source of cholesterol-lowering fiber. Not only do lentils help decrease cholesterol, they are of unique gain in managing blood-sugar problems due to the fact their excessive fiber content prevents blood sugar from rising after a meal. However, this is far from all lentils have to offer. Lentils also provide great amounts of seven essential minerals, B-vitamins, and protein, all without a doubt, no fat. The calorie value of all this nutrition? Just 230 calorie for a whole cup of cooked lentils.

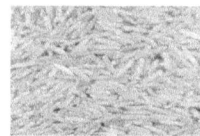 **Brown Rice.**

Brown rice and white rice are totally different from each other! An entire grain of rice has various layers. Only the outermost layer, the hull, is eliminated to produce what we name brown rice. This method is the least unfavorable to the nutritional cost of the rice and avoids the pointless loss of nutrients that takes place within addition processing. If brown rice is milled to get rid of the bran and most of the germ layer, the end result is whiter rice, rice that has lost most of the nutrients. After polishing and sharpening produced white rice, we use to see. Polishing gets rid of the aleurone layer of the grain to extend the shelf lifestyles of the product. The ensuing white rice is clearly a sophisticated starch that is left without its unique nutrients.

Brown rice is an amazing supply of manganese, and a desirable source of selenium, phosphorus, copper, magnesium, and niacin (vitamin B3). All this milling and polishing that converts brown rice into white rice destroys 68% of the vitamin B3, 85% of the vitamin B1, 92% of the vitamin B6, 1/2 of the manganese, more than half of the phosphorus, 65% of the iron, and all of the dietary fiber and crucial fatty acids. By the law in the United States, fully milled and polished white rice must be "enriched" with vitamins B1, B3, and iron. But of course the form of these nutrients when added back into the processed rice is not the same as in the original unprocessed version.

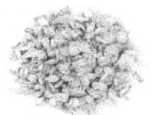

Oats.

Oats are a top-notch supply of manganese and molybdenum. They are additionally a very desirable source of phosphorus as well as a suitable source of copper, biotin, vitamin B1, magnesium, dietary fiber, chromium, zinc, and protein. In the phytonutrient category, oats provide precious quantities of beta-glucans and saponins.

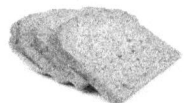

Whole Wheat.

Whole wheat is a very good source of manganese and dietary fiber. It is also a suitable supply of copper, magnesium, and pantothenic acid.

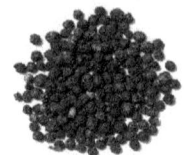

Black Pepper.

As you probably know that black pepper stimulates the taste buds in such a way that an alert is sent to a stomach to increase hydrochloric acid secretion, thereby improving digestion. Hydrochloric acid is essential for the digestion of proteins and different food elements.

Black pepper has long been identified as a carminative, a substance that helps prevent the formation of intestinal gas. On the other hand diuretic promotes urination properties. Black pepper has antioxidant and antibacterial effects it promotes health of the digestive tract. But not only does black pepper helps you get the most benefits of the food, but it also stimulates the breakdown of fats cells, preserving you slim whilst giving you strength.

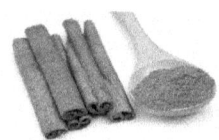

Cinnamon.

Cinnamon's special recuperation capabilities come from three simple kinds of components in the integral oils discovered in its bark. These oils include active components known as cinnamaldehyde, cinnamyl acetate, and cinnamyl alcohol, plus a wide range of different volatile substances.

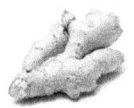

Ginger.

Ginger has a long tradition of being wonderful in assuaging symptoms of gastrointestinal distress. In natural medicine, ginger is considered as a remarkable carminative substance which promotes the removing of intestinal gas and intestinal spasmolytic, a substance which relaxes and soothes the intestinal tract. Much scientific research has shown that ginger possesses numerous therapeutic properties which include antioxidant effects, a potential to inhibit the formation of inflammatory compounds, and direct anti-inflammatory effects.

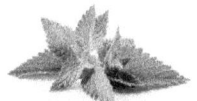

Peppermint.

In the world of health research, randomized managed trials have persistently shown the potential of peppermint oil to relieve signs of irritable bowel syndrome, which include indigestion, dyspepsia, and colonic muscle spasms. These healing properties of peppermint are interestingly related to its clean muscle relaxing ability. Once the easy muscle tissue surrounding the intestine are relaxed, there is much less risk of spasm and indigestion.

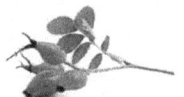

Rose Hip.

Rosehip tea is used to improve and relieve the signs and symptoms of kidney disorders, or to help in the case of slight constipation.

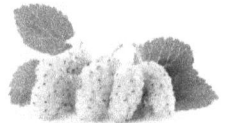

Mulberries.

Mulberries are prosperous in many vitamins and minerals, particularly vitamin C and iron. Vitamin C is an imperative vitamin that is essential for pores and skin health and a number of bodily functions. Iron a vital mineral that has a number of functions, such as transporting oxygen all through your body. Vitamin K1, also recognized as phylloquinone, vitamin K is essential for blood clotting and bone health. Potassium, Vitamin E. Mulberries are additionally packed with antioxidants. Antioxidants are the essential line of defense against free radicals, which shape a dangerous derivative of cellular metabolism that can damage healthful cells, inflicting them to mutate into cancerous ones.

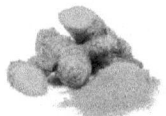

Turmaric.

The active ingredient in turmeric is curcumin, a potent anti-inflammatory that helps maintain healthy inflammation responses. Beneficial in promoting overall joint health and mobility. Promotes Heart Health, Supports overall health of the cardiovascular system.

Encourages Healthy Cholesterol Levels and supports Healthy Metabolism. Aids in maintaining normal blood sugar levels. Optimizes Vitality. Its powerful antioxidant properties fight excess free radicals in the body that can damage cells and diminish health.

Black Seed oil.

Examples of different black seed oil health advantages include: Reducing high blood pressure and excessive cholesterol and improving rheumatoid arthritis symptoms and decreasing asthma symptoms, reducing belly upset. Black seed oil is additionally thought to have anti-cancer properties. It may help fight against pores and skin cancers when applied topically.

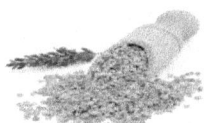

Bee Pollen.

Bee pollen boasts an incredible nutritional profile. It includes over 250 biologically active substances, which includes proteins, carbs, lipids, fatty acids, vitamins, minerals, enzymes, and antioxidants. The high antioxidant content of bee pollen can protect us from chronic diseases, and it can lower heart disease. Could boost body function and protect your liver from toxic substances. May help you avoid illness by way of boosting immunity and killing bacteria. Bee pollen may also have applications for treating and preventing cancers, which appear when cells proliferate abnormally. May ease menopause, which marks the cessation of menstruation in women, that frequently accompanied by using uncomfortable signs such as hot flushes, night sweats, temper changes, and sleep disturbances.

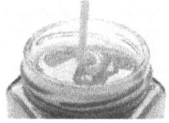 **Raw Honey.**

Raw honey has been used as a people treatment for the duration of history and has a range of health advantages and clinical uses. It's even used in some hospitals as a cure for wounds. Many of these health advantages are particular to raw, or unpasteurized, honey.

Most of the honeys you discover in grocery shops are pasteurized. The excessive warmth kills undesirable yeast, can improve the color and texture, eliminates any crystallization, and extends the shelf life. Many of the really helpful vitamins are also destroyed in the process.

One of the best is Manuka honey, produced in New Zealand through bees that pollinate the Manuka bush; it's one of the most special and really helpful types of honey in the world. Manuka honey uses are, and benefits include: Helps with SIBO, Low stomach acid, Acid reflux. May help treat acne and eczema. Combat infections, treat burns, wounds, and ulcers. It prevents tooth decay and gingivitis. Aids IBS and IBD treatment. Helps to improve sore throats and immunity. Helps allergies, improves sleep.

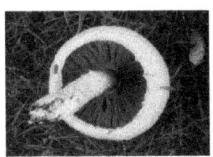 **Mushrooms.**

There are many special types of mushrooms, some of which are fit to be eaten together with typical species such as button, oyster, porcini and chanterelles. There are, however, many species that are not suitable for eating and can in fact cause belly pains or vomiting if eaten, and in some cases could be fatal, such as the common death cap mushroom. So don't ever attempt choosing them for consumption from the woods unless you have been trained to identify them very well. Mushrooms are healthy meals rich in a variety of nutrients. As per USDA mushrooms are an excellent source of minerals and nutritional vitamins that include potassium, phosphorus, magnesium, sodium, vitamin C, niacin, riboflavin, thiamin, folate, and vitamin D.

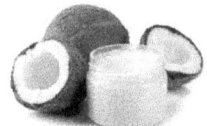 **Coconut oil.**

The health advantages of coconut oil consist of enhancing heart health via increasing the HDL cholesterol levels, promoting weight loss, relieving symptoms of yeast infections, pores and skin, and hair care, improving digestion, and boosting immunity.

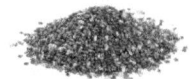 **Chia seeds.**

Chia seeds are amongst the healthiest meals on the planet. They're loaded with nutrients that can have essential benefits for your body and brain. Chia seeds deliver a good amount of nutrients with very low in calories. Chia seeds are good souse of antioxidants and are high in Omega-3 Fatty Acids. Chia seeds are a good source to lower your risk of heart disease. They're high in many important bone nutrients. They also may reduce blood sugar levels and chronic inflammation.

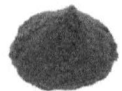

Cocoa Powder.

Cocoa powder is made through crushing cocoa beans and getting rid of the fats or cocoa butter. Cocoa is the richest sources of polyphenols. It's particularly considerable in flavanols, which have strong antioxidant and anti-inflammatory effects. Polyphenols are naturally occurring antioxidants located in fruits, vegetables, tea, chocolate, and wine. They reduce inflammation, better blood flow, lower blood pressure, and improving cholesterol and blood sugar levels. However, processing and heating cocoa can cause it to lose its really useful properties. It's also regularly handled with alkaline to minimize bitterness, which results in a 60% minimize in flavanol content. In addition to lowering blood pressure. Flavanols are involved in the biochemical pathways that produce neurons and necessary molecules for the function of your brain.

CHAPTER VIII
YELLOW PAGES

♦♦♦

Dairy isn't easily classified as healthy or unhealthy because its outcomes may additionally differ significantly between individuals.

There is no compelling proof that humans should keep away from it and lots of evidence of benefits. However, as an infant, your body produced a digestive enzyme known as lactase, which broke down lactose from your mother's milk. However, many humans lose the capacity to break down lactose in adulthood. About 75% of the world's grownup population is unable to break down lactose a phenomenon is known as lactose intolerance.

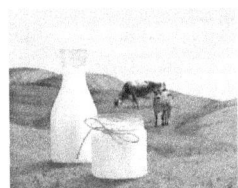 **Cow Milk.**

When acquired from a hundred percent grass-fed cows, whole milk includes a surprising variety of each conventional and phytonutrients. In the traditional category, you'll discover milk to be a very desirable source of vitamin B2 (riboflavin), vitamin D, and vitamin B12. It's also a beneficial supply of the minerals iodine and phosphorus and provides a great amount of calcium. And of course, whole cow's milk is a desirable source of protein.

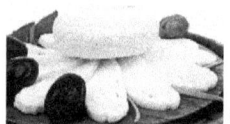**Cheese.**

When produced with whole milk from 100% grass-fed cows, cheese carries a surprising diversity of nutrients—not merely protein and calcium as many people might assume. Whole-milk grass-fed cheese furnishes measurable quantities of 4 essential fat-soluble vitamins: A, D, E, and K. They also grant antioxidant vitamins like selenium, zinc, and beta-carotene, as well as all B-complex vitamins, which include B1, B2, B3, B5, B6, B12, choline, and biotin. Whole-milk grass-fed cheese additionally grants essential fats like omega-3s and CLA, as well as a health-promoting ratio of omega-6: omega-3 fat. There are surely few meals that offer this identical variety of nutrients. For example, nuts and seeds can provide many of the equal fat-related nutrients while vegetables can supply many of the same antioxidants in even more plentiful amounts.

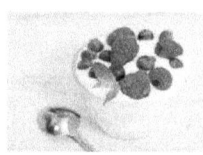**Grass-Fed Yogurt.**

Grass-fed yogurt offers CLA (conjugated linoleic acid), a health-supportive fatty acid is regularly absent from non-grass-fed yogurts. Grass-fed yogurt is a very desirable source of iodine, vitamin B12, phosphorus, and calcium. It is additionally a suitable supply of vitamin B2, molybdenum, pantothenic acid, protein, zinc, and biotin.

If digestive benefits are amongst your top motives for thinking about the inclusion of yogurt in your meal plan, I suggest a selection of yogurts clearly labeled to have one million or other active bacterial cultures (CFUs). However, I also believe that grass-fed, cow's milk yogurt can supply you with vital health advantages even if the quantity of active bacteria in the yogurt is a lot smaller.

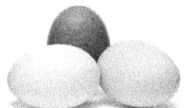 **Eggs.**

The predominant motive eggs had been regarded to be unhealthy in the past, is that the yolks are high in cholesterol.

Cholesterol is a waxy substance discovered in food, and it is additionally made through your body. Many years ago, comprehensive research linked eggs to high blood cholesterol and heart disease.

In 1961, the American Heart Association encouraged limiting dietary cholesterol. Many other global health organizations did the same. However, there are also advantages of consuming egg. Eggs have long been identified as a supply of remarkable protein. World Health Organization and some other public health authorities use egg as a reference standard to evaluate protein quality in all different foods. Egg protein is typically referred to as "HBV" protein, which means protein with High Biological Value.

All B vitamins are discovered in eggs, which includes vitamins B1, B2, B3, B5, B6, B12, including choline, biotin, and folic acid.

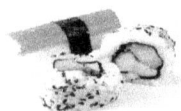
Sushi.

Sushi is made of the white rice, and it's considered as a high-glycemic food with very little protein that can result in fast increases in blood sugar and insulin levels.

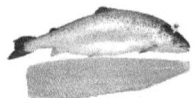
Salmon.

The unique protein and amino acid composition of salmon are frequently overlooked in its nutritional profile. Salmon carries short protein molecules called peptides that have been proven to be bioactive and essential anti-inflammatory properties. Salmon also provides necessary amounts of the antioxidant amino acid taurine. Salmon is a fantastic supply of vitamin B12, vitamin D, and selenium. It's a great source of niacin, omega-3 fatty acids, protein, phosphorus, and vitamin B6. It is additionally an excellent source of choline, pantothenic acid, biotin, and potassium.

In another hand, the study shows that fish-derived Omega-3s increased of colon cancer metastasis compared to a low-fat diet. And if you're worried about bone density than forget salmon: Because fish has highly-acidic flesh which speeds calcium loss and also contributes to osteoporosis and kidney stones. In any case, of course, wild salmon is far healthier than its farmed relative. In case you eat farmed salmon, you're asking for trouble because farm-raised salmon contains unhealthy levels of contaminants so-called PCBs, polychlorinated biphenyls. PCBs are industrial products and chemicals, dioxins. Chemicals that cause cancer developmental problems in children.

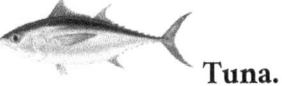 **Tuna.**

Tuna is an excellent supply of selenium, vitamin B3 (niacin), vitamin B12, vitamin B6, and protein. It is a very desirable source of phosphorus as well as a suitable source of vitamin B1 (thiamin), vitamin B2 (riboflavin), choline, vitamin D, and the minerals potassium, iodine, and magnesium. Some of the selenium is located in the structure of selenoneine, which is very good for its antioxidant properties. In addition, tuna offers precious quantities of omega-3 fatty acids (including eicosapentaenoic acid or EPA, and docosahexaenoic acid or DHA.

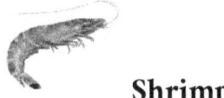 **Shrimp.**

Shrimp is a unique supply of the carotenoid astaxanthin. It's also a superb supply of selenium and vitamin B12. This shellfish is a very desirable source of protein, including phosphorus, as well as choline, copper, and iodine. Also, it is a good source of all B-complex vitamins, as well as vitamin A and vitamin E. Shrimp additionally ranks as a suitable supply of omega-3 fatty acids and includes roughly equal quantities of two unique Omega-3s, EPA (eicosapentaenoic acid) and DHA (docosahexaenoic acid). Shrimp is additionally a desirable source of the mineral zinc.

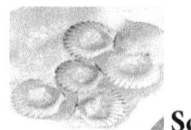
⊿ Scallops.

Scallops contain a range of vitamins that can promote your cardiovascular health, plus provide safety against colon cancer.

Scallops are an incredible source of vitamin B12 and phosphorus. They are additionally an excellent source of protein, selenium, and choline as well as a top source of zinc, magnesium, and potassium.

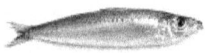
Sardines.

Sardines are rich in several vitamins that have been discovered to guide cardiovascular health. They are one of the best sources of the omega-3 fatty acids EPA and DHA. One serving 100 grams can of sardines contains over 50% of the daily value for these necessary nutrients. Sardines are a top-notch supply of vitamin B12, ranking as one of the World's Healthiest Food most focused on this nutrient. Vitamin B12 promotes cardiovascular well-being due to the fact it is intricately tied to maintaining levels of homocysteine in balance; homocysteine can harm artery walls, with elevated levels being a risk aspect for atherosclerosis. They are an excellent source of phosphorus, omega-3 fatty acids, protein, and vitamin D. additionally; they are an excellent source of calcium, niacin, copper, vitamin B2, and choline.

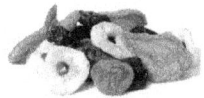 **Dried Fruit.**

Food carries calories and consuming too many calories-even of wholesome foods-leads to weight gain. But there are healthy energy and unhealthy "empty" calories, and fruit is a good source of calories. But because dried fruit is much smaller than the fresh fruit from which it comes, it is less complicated to eat and adds a lot of calories by consuming dried fruit. Another count of the problem is that some dried fruit makers add sugars to dried fruit, which already include their very own natural sugars.

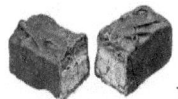 **Protein Bars.**

When you are on the run and don't have time to put together a healthful meal or snack, protein bars can be a handy substitute. The excessive protein content helps maintain you full, and the added vitamins and minerals can also cover viable deficiencies in your diet. But we should consider that many protein bars contain added sugars and synthetic components. Furthermore, you are very likely to get too much of some vitamins and minerals and miss out on the health advantages of whole meals if you consume more than one/two bars a day. Your protein bar consumption shouldn't substitute a balanced food plan of fruit and vegetables.

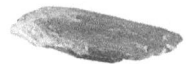

Grass-Fed Beef.

Yes, Beef is a source of vitamin B12 and source of protein, niacin, vitamin B6, selenium, zinc, and phosphorus. It is additionally an excellent source of choline, pantothenic acid, iron, potassium, and vitamin B2 but having said that Eating beef product is a unique way to expand your waistline and increase your possibilities of becoming unhealthy and develop heart disease, diabetes, arthritis, and other health conditions. Research has shown that vegetarians have a forty percent less cancer rate than meat-eaters. Plus, meat-eaters are nine times greater likely to be obese than vegans are. Remember that when you eat animal-derived foods, antibiotics, dioxins, and a lot of different toxics will most likely accumulate in your body and stay there for years.

Cows are gentle social animals. They can recognize more than one hundred different cows, and they structure close friendships with members of their family and friends. Researchers report that cows grieve when their buddies or household members die.

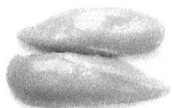

Chicken.

Chicken offers omega-3 fatty acids, inclusive of each EPA (eicosatetraenoic acid) and DHA (docosahexaenoic acid). Except for biotin (which is still quite controversial as an element of rooster meat), chicken additionally offers measurable quantities of all B vitamins. Chicken is a first-rate source of niacin. It is additionally an excellent supply of protein, selenium, vitamin B6, phosphorus, choline, pantothenic acid, and vitamin B12.

Certified organic is the best you can purchase from the supermarket, and it is pricey, in part due to the fact it means no drugs, antibiotics, chemical additives, or pesticides.

Free-range means that chickens go outside fenced aria every day, although there's no requirement to how long they spend outdoors.

Raised without antibiotics doesn't mean drug-free — these chickens are allowed to be dosed with different meds.

Raised without hormones is a label you might also regularly see. However, it's pretty meaningless, as the USDA doesn't permit their use in chicken in the first place. Hormones are regularly used in Beef.

Natural or farm-raised are pretty useless terms, which inform buyers nothing about the way the chicken was once raised, what it was fed, or if it was treated with meds and antibiotics. In fact, your chickens going to China to be cooked, packaged, and then returned to the U.S or elsewhere for sale.

Given China's questionable track report on food safety, this seems like one of the most wasteful and probably dangerous chicken-processing schemes ever devised. I urge you to battle back via refusing to purchase frozen, pre-cooked, ready-to-serve, or heat and eat processed chicken products.

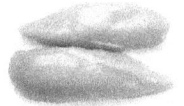 **Turkey.**

Turkey perhaps has the best protein. Skinned turkey breast offers about 34 grams of protein in a 4-ounce serving. This food ranks as a very suitable source of protein in our meals ranking system. All B nutritional vitamins are present in turkey meat, which include B1, B2, B3, B5, B6, B12, folate, biotin, and choline. (However, because the biotin content of turkey meat is sensitive to the turkey's dietary intake, the quantity of this nutrition can range significantly.) In terms of our ranking system, turkey is a very suitable supply of vitamins B1, B2, B3, B6, and also its source of choline.

Advantages of the food shown on yellow pages are the satisfactory version of the product we can consume, but I have listed them on yellow pages, here is why:

World Health Organization declared processed meat a 'carcinogen' which will increase one's risk of colon or rectum cancer with the aid of 18 percent. But it's no longer processed meat that places you at risk. A tremendous array of studies from top universities and independent researchers has discovered that consuming chicken, cow, and other animals promote cancer in many forms. Extensive research in England and Germany showed that vegetarians had been about 40 percent less in all likelihood to enhance most cancers in contrast to meat-eaters, the most common varieties being breast, prostate, and colon cancers. Harvard study discovered that just one serving a day of red meat during childhood was related with a 22 percent higher hazard of pre-menopausal breast cancer and that the equal red meat consumption in adulthood was related with a thirteen percent higher risk of breast cancer overall.

A wide variety of hypotheses are used to explain the connection between meat consumption and most cancers risk. First, meat is devoid of fiber and different nutrients that have a protective impact against cancer. Meat also includes animal protein, saturated fat, and, in some cases, carcinogenic compounds such as heterocyclic amines (HCA) and polycyclic aromatic hydrocarbons (PAH), which are formed during the processing or cooking. Meat additionally contains hormones, which expand your cancer risk. Cows grow at an unnaturally quick rate because the cattle industry feeds them pellets full of hormones. While low ranges of naturally-occurring hormones are found in several foods, many scientists are worried that the artificial hormones injected into cows notably cause health issues in humans who consume them. And while organic or hormone-free meat might be a better option, you still not eliminating your chances of consuming the naturally-occurring sex hormones existing in the animals when they were killed. The sex hormones progesterone, testosterone, and estrogen are all naturally occurring in animals, whether or not they've been given synthetic hormones or not, so when you consume those animals, you are additionally consuming hormones.

After fully reviewing the collected scientific literature, a Working Group of 22 experts from 10 countries convened by means of the IARC Monographs Programme classified the consumption of red meat as probably carcinogenic to human beings (Group 2A), based on limited evidence that the consumption of red meat causes most cancers in human beings and strong mechanistic evidence supporting a carcinogenic effect.

This association was once observed mainly for colorectal cancer. However, associations were also viewed for pancreatic cancer and prostate cancer.

Processed meat.

Processed meat was once labeled as carcinogenic to human beings (Group 1), based on sufficient evidence in people who consume processed meat causes colorectal cancer.

Meat consumption and its effects: The use of meat varies significantly between countries, with from a few percent's up to a hundred percent of people, eating red meat, depending on the country, and somewhat decrease proportions consuming processed meat.

The professionals concluded that each 50-gram portion of processed meat eaten day by day would increase the chance of colorectal cancer by 19%. However, for an individual's developing colorectal cancer because of their consumption of processed meat remains small, but of course, this threat will increase with the amount of meat consumed.

Because of the broad range of humans who consume processed meat, the international effect on cancer incidence is public health importance. The most interesting evidence came from large studies conducted over the previous 20 years.

These findings further aid current public health guidelines to restriction the consumption of meat.

When I say red meat, I mean all types of meat, such as Beef, veal, pork, lamb, mutton, horse, goat, and so on including chicken and fish.

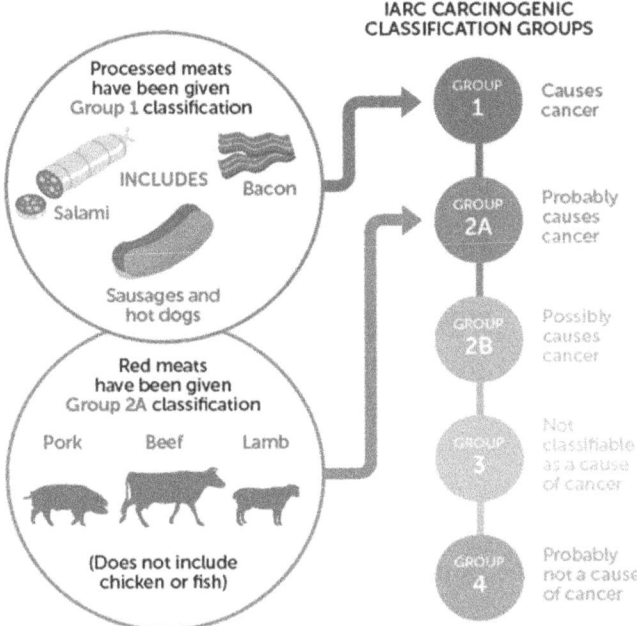

These categories represent how likely something is to cause cancer in humans, not how many cancers it causes.

As we all know, processed meat refers to meat that has been modified by salting, curing, fermentation, smoking, or other techniques to enhance flavor or improve preservation. Most processed meats include pork or Beef. However, processed meats may additionally include different red meats, poultry, offal, fish, etc.

CHAPTER IX
RED PAGES

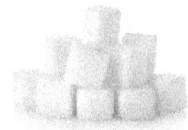

Sugar.

Sugar promotes wrinkling and aging skin, additionally Makes blood acidic, it can lead to osteoporosis. Can rot your teeth, raises your blood sugar level, Contributes to obesity, it's addictive almost as a much as drugs, it provides 'empty calories' and of course it has no nutritional value what so ever. It contributes to diabetes and robs your body of essential minerals, robs of your energy, and contributes to heart diseases. It can cause cancer and contribute to ulcers, can cause gallstones and contribute to adrenal fatigue. Sugar can suppress your immune system, Raises the level of neurotransmitters called serotonin, Weakens eyesight. It's very impotent to look at Labels on the back of the packaging and read information.

While this does no longer tell you the number of free sugars, it is a beneficial way of comparing labels. Select ingredients that are lower in sugar.

Products are regarded to both be high or low in sugar if they fall above or below the following thresholds:

high: more than 23.5g of total sugars per 100g

low: 4g or less of total sugars per 100g

If the quantity of sugars per 100g is between these figures, it is considered as a medium level.

The sugar figure describes the total quantity of sugars from all sources of free sugars, plus from milk, fruit, and vegetables.

For example, simple yogurt might also include as much as 8g per serving, but none of these are free sugars, because they all come from milk.

Apple may include around 10g of total sugar, depending on the size of the fruit selected variety and of course stage of ripeness.

But sugar in fruit is not regarded as free sugars except the fruit is juiced or pureed.

This means meals containing fruit or milk will be a healthier choice than one containing loads of free sugars, even if two products contain the same total quantity of sugar.

You can tell if the food carries a lot of added sugars via checking the elements list.

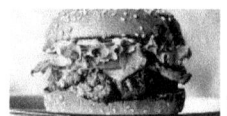 **Burgers.**

If you consume more calories than you can expend you will gain weight and burgers can be high-calorie foods. A double hamburger with mayonnaise carries 943 calories. Burgers are high in cholesterol and saturated fat. Dietary cholesterol and saturated fats can elevate levels of cholesterol in your blood and accordingly increase your chance for heart disease. A double hamburger with mayo includes 23 grams of saturated fat, or 109 % of the daily value, and 173 milligrams of cholesterol, or 58 % of the daily value based on a 2,000-calorie diet. Also, burgers can be high in sodium, with a double hamburger with mayo containing 1,082 milligrams. A small one-patty burger except mayo has 259 milligrams of sodium. A high-sodium diet is a very unhealthy choice; it can lead to high blood pressure and very likely to increase the risk of heart diseases, stroke, and kidney diseases. Healthy adults have to eat no more than 2,300 milligrams of sodium per day.

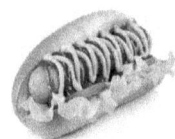 **Sausage.**

The things that are inflicting all the fuss are chemical compounds known as nitrites and nitrates that are found in sausage which once in the body can be converted into cancer-causing compounds. The accordance of a spokesman for Cancer Research UK, these matters appear naturally in red meat. However, there are additionally often added at some stage in meat-processing as a preservative. All red meat includes a red pigment referred to as haems, as soon as in the gut, it can be broken down to form N-nitroso compounds, or NOCs, many of which are regarded to cause cancer. Additionally, haems might also irritate or damage the cells lining the bowel, which can lead to them dividing more rapidly, sort of action is more likely to increase the danger of developing cancer. The aggregate of the two, as well as sausages' pretty high fats and salt content, which have additionally been linked to increased dangers of developing cancer, has led to a recommendation to reduce both processed and red meat.

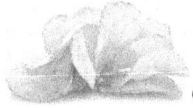 **Chips.**

There has been much research and concluded that consuming a packet of chips can develop into a chance of heart disease, most cancers in adults, obesity, and most importantly, it can become very addictive for children. Chips can be high in fat, sugar, and salt, especially in the salt, there is a lot of salt in every packet of chips which can lead to obesity, type-2 diabetes, and coronary disease. If you are consuming a lot of quantity of chips each day, this could have harmful outcomes on unborn babies. Poisonous chemical compounds are existing in the snacks that are known as ACRYLAMIDE. It is odorless, tasteless, and invisible, however, can prove to be hazardous to DNA. It is a nerve poison that first found in plastics and dyeing industries. The oil used for fry potato chips is fat which includes excessive levels of cholesterol. Most of the potatoes are deep-fried in oil. High levels of oil can increase the chance of high blood pressure. They commonly have a hundred and twenty and 180 milligrams of sodium per ounce. So human beings are ingesting extra sodium and fats without even realizing it.

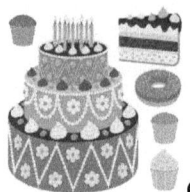 **Cake.**

In short, the cakes are not healthy! However, some cakes are much less unhealthy than others, and if you make your cakes, maybe you can make some changes just to enhance their nutritional profile.

One serving, 8-inch cake, contains 249 calories even without frosting. Top it with three tablespoons of chocolate frosting, and you are adding another 164 calories. If you eat 2,000 calories per day, it's about one-fourth of your calories for the day. That slice of cake additionally carries 10 grams of fat, which include 2.8 grams of saturated fat. If you add chocolate frosting, it will contribute another 7.3 grams of fat and 2.4 grams of saturated fat. This combination in total will be 27 percent of the DV for total fats and 26 percent of the DV for saturated fat. Just 2/3 tablespoons of frosting include almost the whole day's allowance for added sugar for women, providing 23.8 of the 26-gram, the sugar limit recommended by the American Heart Association as a recommended limit for men is 37.5 grams. When we eat the cake that goes with the frosting, and you will have eaten up an unhealthy amount of added sugar. Healthy people limit their sodium consumption to no more than 2,300 milligrams per day because excessive amounts of sodium can make a contribution to high blood pressure and increase your heart disease risk. One slice of cake contains 235 milligrams of sodium, and if we add chocolate frosting, it could contribute another 76 milligrams, for a total of 310 milligrams, or 14 percent of the recommended limit.

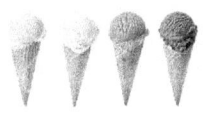 **Ice Cream.**

For some people, Ice cream is one of the most desirable foods on earth. Unfortunately, ice cream is also one of the unhealthiest. Most commercial ice creams are full of sugar. It's also high in calories, and it is very easy to eat excessive amounts. Eating it for dessert is even worse, due to the fact then you include it all on top of your total calorie intake.

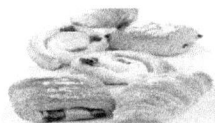 **Pastries.**

The most pastries, cookies, and cakes are extremely unhealthy. They are commonly made with refined sugar, including refined wheat flour plus added fats, that are often disturbingly unhealthy fats, high in trans fats. These tasty treats are some of the worst things that you can put into your body: almost no essential nutrients, but lots of calories and unhealthy ingredients.

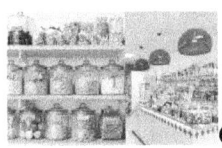 **Candy Bars.**

Candy bars are also very unhealthy. They are excessive in sugar, added refined wheat flour including processed fat. They are, of course, very low in essential nutrients. Processed foods like candy bars are commonly engineered to be super tasty (so you consume more) and have been designed so that it is very effortless to consume them quickly. A sweet bar may additionally taste excellent and cause some temporary satiety, but you'll be hungry again very rapidly because of the way these poisonous-sugar treats are metabolized. I would suggest you eat a piece of fruit instead, or a piece of actual high-cocoa dark chocolate.

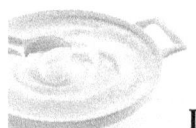

Low-Fat Yogurt.

Most yogurts found in the grocery stores are awful for you. They are often low in fat, however, loaded with sugar to make up for the lack of taste that the fats provided. In most cases the yogurt has had the healthy, natural dairy fats removed, only to be replaced with something much worse. Additionally, many yogurts don't genuinely contain probiotic bacteria, as usually believed. The yogurts have often been pasteurized, after fermentation, which kills all the bacteria. Alternatives: Choose regular, full-fat yogurt that includes live or active cultures (probiotics). If you love yogurt, try to get yogurt from grass-fed cows.

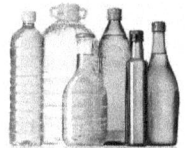

Refined Vegetable Oil.

Now day's humans have increased their consumption of added fats. However, this drastically increases in the consumption of unhealthy vegetable oils, such as soybean oil, corn oil, including cottonseed oil and canola oil. These oils are very excessive in omega-6 fatty acids, which people never consumed in such massive quantities before. There are many serious issues with these oils. They are exceptionally sensitive to oxidation and cause increased oxidative stress in the body. They also can increase the risk of cancer. Alternatives: Use healthier fats like coconut oil, extra virgin olive oil, or avocado oil instead.

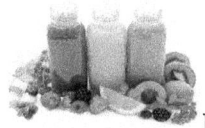 **Fruit Juice.**

We often assume that Fruit juice is healthy. However, this is a mistake. Usually, many fruit juices are little more than fruit-flavored sugar water. Yes, juice contains some antioxidants and vitamin C, but this has to be weighed against the large quantity of liquid sugar. Fruit juice contains simply as plenty of sugar as a sugary drink like Coke or Lemonade, and sometimes even more. There are some alternatives; the best way is to buy juicer or blender and make yourself vegetable or fruit juice at home without adding extra sugar. However, these should be regarded as supplement, not something you drink every day to quench thirst. Drink water instead.

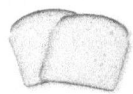 **Bread.**

Bread is normally made from wheat, and it contains the protein gluten, and even only for this reason, all wheat-based bread is not good for those who have celiac disease and or those who have gluten sensitivity. Furthermore most commercial breads are unhealthy, even for a human who do tolerate gluten. This is due to the fact the great majority of them are made from refined wheat, which is low in essential vitamins (empty calories) and leads to rapid spikes in blood sugar. Alternatives: For humans who can tolerate gluten, Ezekiel bread is a great choice. Whole grain bread is additionally really better than white bread.

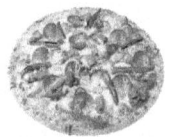 **Pizza.**

Pizza is one of the world's most famous junk foods. This is no longer surprising, given that it tastes brilliant and is quite handy to eat. The trouble is that most commercially prepared pizzas are made with critically unhealthy ingredients most of the times. The dough is usually made from refined wheat flour which is unhealthy, and the meat on top of it is generally processed. Pizza is also extremely high in calories. Alternatives: Some pizza places use more healthy ingredients. Homemade pizzas can additionally be healthier, as long as you pick healthy ingredients.

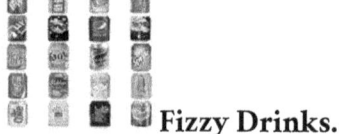 **Fizzy Drinks.**

We all know that some sources of sugar are worse than others, and sugary drinks are the absolute worst. When humans drink sugar calories, the brain does not register them as food. For this reason, humans do not mechanically compensate through consuming less of different ingredients instead, and end up significantly increasing their total calorie intake. When consumed in large amounts of sugar can drive insulin resistance in the body and is strongly linked to non-alcoholic fatty liver disease. It is additionally related to various diseases, including of diabetes and heart disease. Sugary drinks are also the most fattening thing of the modern diet, and drinking them in massive quantities can drive fat gain and obesity.

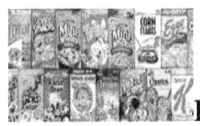

Breakfast Cereals.

It disgraces the way some breakfast cereals are marketed. Many of them, which include those that are marketed towards children, have all varieties of health claims plastered on the box. This also includes misleading things such as whole grain or low fat. But when you genuinely look at the ingredients list, you see that it's nearly nothing however refined grains, sugar, and artificial chemicals. The fact is if the packaging of food says that it is healthy, and then it likely isn't. The healthy foods are those that do not need any health claims, whole single-ingredient foods. Real meals do not even need an ingredients list because real food IS the ingredient.

Processed Cheese.

Processed cheese products are a scam; they are nothing like regular cheese. They are generally made with filler components that are combined and engineered to have a comparable appear and texture as cheese. Carefully read labels, and make sure that the cheese you're ingesting is actually a cheese.

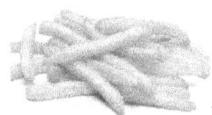

French Fries.

Did you know that even a small serving of French fries from famous fast food shops carries between 200 and 340 calories on average? But who eats small servings anymore? If you order large fries, you end up getting between 371 and 735 calories. In those calories, there is typically between 8 and 18 grams of fat, with around 1.5 to 3.5 grams of saturated fats for a small fries serving. Large fries have between eleven and a massive 37 grams of fat, with 4.5 grams of saturated fat. French fries served in restaurants frequently come dipped in corn oil even earlier than they are fried. Processed corn oil is regarded as one of the worst types of oils for our body. Corn oil has 70 times more inflammatory omega-6 fatty acids than Omega-3s.

The foods that have been fried in hydrogenated vegetable oils like corn, canola, and soybean oil are especially damaging to our health. The polyunsaturated fats, they comprise, become contaminated, with the constant heating and reheating, which of course degrades their structure in general. These extremely unhealthy heat damaged fats are strongly implicated in promoting inflammation inside our body that is often starting point of many common health problems and diseases.

Next time you stroll past a small, fast food area try and have a look at where these French fries are cooked. Have a look dirty brown color and consistency of that oil as it is heated over and over again. Would you drink a cup of it? Well, it seems many humans are, each and every week in the French fries they eat.

So far, the simplest and best way to eat healthily and lose weight is to keep away from processed foods as much as you can. All Fizzy drinks. Chocolates. Sweets. Mass-produced bread. Chicken nuggets. Reconstituted meat products along with most sausages. Powdered soup. Margarine. Biscuits. Breakfast cereal. Energy bars. Energy drinks. Flavored milk. Ready meals with ready-made sauces. Powdered slimming products. Pre-prepared pies.

Simply if it appears like it was made in a factory, then it is likely bad for you.

And let me remind you again the good rule to bear in mind is that a real meal doesn't need an ingredients list, due to the fact actual meal is an ingredient. This is some of the food images below that we should avoid at all cost

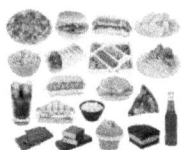 — **Pizza, Hot dog, Breakfast cereals, Chocolates, Cookies, Fizzy drinks, etc.**

CHAPTER X
REUSABLE PLASTIC CUPS AND FOOD CONTAINERS

♦ ♦ ♦

You probably have heard about BPA and obscurely recognize your water bottle shouldn't have it. Have you ever questioned if different plastics are safe, or if it's genuinely worth it to keep away from plastic containers?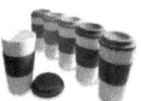

Finding solutions to these questions can be quite severe. The FDA also says plastic, and the things that make them, like BPA and phthalates, are safe, but research is continuously coming out pointing out the opposite. Anyway, how does plastic get into our food? We keep meals in plastic, prepare it on plastic, and cook dinner in plastic, so there are a lot of factors of contact that can cause what is called leaching or migration of chemical compounds from plastic to food. The research shows that no food container is free from leaching, although leaching can be extra frequent and hazardous from some types of plastic packaging than others like glass.

Food can be a relatively risky substance: Acids in meals like lemons and tomatoes can corrode containers. Additionally, fats and oils can cause the plastic to leach more quickly. Soda erodes your teeth, so think about what it could do to a piece of plastic? Heated plastic leaches chemical substances fifty five times faster, so whether you're reheating a plastic plate in the microwave, putting warm meals in a storage container, or using a plate that's been run thru a warm dishwasher, you're at risk of chemical leaching.

Let's talk about BPA and phthalates, what are they?

There are many sorts of plastics. Particular substances are often added to plastic to help structure it, stabilize it, and change its flexibility.

You've likely heard about BPA bisphenol-A, a substance added to plastic to shape polycarbonate plastics - a popular kind of plastic due to the fact it's transparent, rigid, heat-resistant and very hard to break. Phthalates are some other common substance added to plastics to make them soft and flexible. Anyway just like plastic, BPA is everywhere we go. Polycarbonate "Group of thermoplastic polymers containing carbonate groups in their chemical structures" plastics, that are made using BPA, are used in everything from so-called reusable water bottles, including plastic plates and food storage containers and even the receipt you snatch at the grocery store. Even metal cans are lined with BPA-based liners so meals can't damage metal cans. BPA is also used on many paper cups to hold your coffee and tea from leaking. You can look for the code on the bottom of a container. If it has a number from three to 8, it may contain BPA. A national survey, NHANES, discovered that 93% of people six years and older had BPA in their urine.

Phthalates are a group of chemical substances discovered in a vast, broad array of products, and it can be challenging to recognize if they're in any given one. Phthalate is everywhere. It can be found in the air we breathe, in the dust of our homes, in the drugs, including cosmetics and water. Phthalates are used in thousands of products, like toys, detergents, even in blood bags, and personal care products. Since 2008, some varieties of phthalates have been eliminated from children's toys, and some nations have gone further and entirely rightly banned them

When you are trying to avoid plastics with phthalates watch out for polyvinyl chloride, PVC, or the number 3 on the backside of the package. While the Fair Packaging and Labeling Act (FPLA) requires phthalates to be labeled on a box, it is not required to be labeled if it's in the structure of fragrance. Due to this, many people who attempt to keep away from phthalates chose to purchase packaging without added fragrance.

Why is plastic so dangerous?

Plastics are all examined and are expected to be stable throughout day-to-day use. The FDA considers BPA to be safe. It's estimated that the average daily consumption of BPA is 4000 times less than the U.S. Environmental Protection Agency finds acceptable. It also considers the health consequences of phthalates to be negligible.

On the other hand, research has discovered all kinds of strange things to be related to revealing the BPA. Did you know that BPA and phthalates can mimic human hormones? That is why they are referred to as (endocrine disruptors). The endocrine system impacts a massive group of activities in your body such as metabolism, growth, reproduction, immunity, and sleep - all systems you want to work at 100%. While stages of these chemical substances discovered within people are thought to be at kind of acceptable and safe levels, lots of research over the last few years find the opposite.

However, in the case of plastic labeled BPA-free, is it safe? One latest study bought over 450 products from a range of stores like

Walmart and Whole Foods. They then put them via normal wear and tear by dishwashing, microwaving and also exposing them to sunlight and found that more than 95% of these plastics, which had all been labeled as BPA-free, emitted chemical compounds that acted like estrogen, simply like BPA. Therefore while we believe that BPA is on its way out, the reality is that the replacements to BPA haven't been studied as well and may also have similar effects. In fact, BPS, a famous plastic substitute for BPA in water bottles, does not have to be labeled at all and once ingested behaves much the same way as BPA.

What are some potential health effects?

One of the motives we can't say for sure that these chemicals are dangerous is due to how difficult it can be to test. Experiments are carried out on animals, which have slightly different metabolisms and reactions than our own. In human trials, much of the research carried out is in massive population research rather than the more definitive managed trials. You can't lock a human in a plastic-free world - take into account it's everywhere. Other study notes that there is no database for the BPA content material in foods, making it difficult to calculate everyday exposure and publicity overtime effectively.

BPA and different hormone disruptors like phthalates have been linked to higher blood pressure (within hours of ingesting from plastic vs. a glass cup), obesity, diabetes, and inflammatory bowel disease. It can also cause early puberty and limit sperm counts and fertility.

Hormone disruptors can be in particular worrisome for developing fetuses. One study discovered that when BPA was passed from the mom throughout pregnancy, it caused inflammation alongside the digestive tract and liver, which can be a sign of chronic inflammation. They additionally noted the microorganism found in the gut was once altered, and we understand such adjustments have been linked from the entirety from allergies to depression to weight gain. Another study discovered a connection between autism and BPA.

This list is by no means comprehensive. But in a way, does it need to be? We understand that plastic does leach from containers. We know that BPA appears to be doing something, as does its replacements. And both ways, we can do something about it, by using the products that aren't made of or lined with plastic. So what can you do to keep away from BPA and different plastics?

We can switch from a reusable plastic bottle to one made from stainless steel or glass.

On the go cups? If you're like me you possibly thought to grab a paper cup was once better for you and the environment however sorry folks - paper cups are also often lined with BPA. Okay, where is the solution? Carry your personal stainless steel mug. (I see people bringing their metal mugs in coffee shops!)

What about canned goods? Buy fresh and frozen fruits and veggies as an alternative to canned goods.

Try to ignore taking a receipt. Many are lined with BPA.

We should avoid plastic wraps and use glass storage containers instead.

What about the microwave? Make sure to place meals on a glass or ceramic plate before reheating.

Can we use plastic for storage? No, Consider recycling your plastic Tupperware and use glass containers.

Unfortunately, warm water goes passed a lot of plastic in most coffee machines. Consider the use of a French press.

CHAPTER XI
MINDFULNESS

Mindfulness is awareness. It means paying attention in the present moment, to maintain awareness of our thoughts, feelings, and bodily sensations. Some of you who haven't experienced have never tried on; you may ask legitimate questions to what is mindfulness? In a brief description, the mindfulness is the quality or state of being conscious or aware of something, peacefully focusing on awareness on the present moment. Mindfulness means understanding what is going on inside and outside of ourselves, moment by moment.

It's very easy to stop noticing the world around you. It's additionally easy to lose touch with our bodies and feeling and to end up living in our head, caught up in our thoughts without stopping to observe how these thoughts are driving our emotions and behavior.

An essential section of mindfulness is reconnecting with our bodies and the sensations we experience. It means waking up to the sights, sounds, smells, and tastes of the present moment.

Another crucial phase of mindfulness is an awareness of our thoughts and feelings as they occur from moment to moment.

We have to allow our self to see the present moment. If we manage to do that, it can positively change the way we see our self's and our life.

The mindfulness helps intellectual well-being. If you become more aware of the present moment, it will help you enjoy the world around you greater and understand yourself better.

When we develop to be more conscious of the current moment, we commence seeing sparkling things that we have been taking for granted.

Mindfulness additionally will help us to emerge as more conscious of the movement of thoughts and feelings that we experience. See how we can develop to be entangled in that movement in methods that are no longer helpful.

This lets us stand back from our ideas and begin to see their patterns. Gradually, we can teach ourselves to observe when our ideas are taking over and understand that thoughts are mental activities that do not have to manage us.

Most of us have issues that we discover challenging to let go, so mindfulness can aid us to deal with them more productively.

Awareness of this type additionally helps us be conscious signs and symptoms of stress or anxiety beforehand and helps us deal with them better.

There is a way to how to be more mindful, reminding yourself to be conscious of your thoughts, feelings, physique sensations, and the world around you is the first step to mindfulness.

Even as we go about our day by day lives, we can phrase the sensations of things, the meals we eat, the air moving past the body as we walk, All this may sound very small, however it has massive power to interrupt the autopilot mode we generally interact day today, and to provide us new views on life. While in mindfulness, every thought, feeling, and sensation that arises automatically enters into this challenge and, this is the necessary part; we can gently acknowledge and acquaint as it is and without judging it in any way.

If this is difficult to imagine, don't worry. For most of this nonjudgmental consciousness happens itself when you exercise correctly. The essential element to take into account, for now, is that mindfulness is not a rejection of anything.

Mindfulness is an open acceptance of the entirety that comes into your awareness. If you're working towards conscious breathing, don't reject thoughts that come into your mind simply due to the fact they interrupt your mindful breathing. Observing these thoughts, which are commonly ignored, then again continuously dispersing our awareness and coloring our perception, is an essential phase of working in the direction of mindfulness. So this is perfectly fine.

Simply properly acknowledge the thinking in mindfulness, actually as you had been doing with your breath, and then let the idea pass. Then carry your focal point back to your breath. As time goes on, your ability to pay attention to one aspect for a length of time as well as your ability to observe things with your mindfulness will improve. And with it, the greater of your mindfulness practice will improve as well. Just being capable of acknowledging when your thoughts stray will take some time. In the beginning, your exercise will appear and experience like this:

Just concentrate on your breath. Lose focus inside a few seconds, aware of the thought or feeling you strayed too, however most of the time not. Back to concentrating on your breath. That's it. But after a while, you'll start to be aware these thoughts and emotions often increased, more clearly, and that will allow you to be renowned them with your mindfulness.

There is more than one way to practice mindfulness, to talk more about mindfulness its exercise and influences, but the thing is that the point of the teaching is to provide you right path and tips. Considering the size of the paragraph as it must be uncomplicated to carry on you everywhere you go, that's because it should be practical and more useful. Once you start practicing mindfulness, meditation, and yoga, you will discover loads of information on YouTube, and on the route, there are plenty of books available as well which will help you achieve your goal.

CHAPTER XII
MEDITATION
♦ ♦ ♦

Meditation is a training of the mind to withdraw the thoughts from the automated responses to sense-impressions, and to lead to a state of ideal patience and attention, the potential to go beyond the barriers of the physical body and the mind. Meditation is to focus strongly on one point and continually bring your attention back to that focal point when it wanders. Some of the reasons why most human being who has tried Meditation have concluded that it's very challenging is because they are making an attempt to do the Meditation. You can't do Meditation; however, you can become meditative. So it is not a thing that you can do. Nobody can do Meditation. However, you can grow to be meditative. Meditation is a certain quality. It is not a specific act. If you prepare your body, your mind, your energies, and your feelings to a particular stage, Meditation will naturally flower inside you. It is a joyful feeling that one can experience inside himself.

If you maintain the body still, the mind will also naturally come to be still. I want you to look at yourself and see how many needless moves your body makes when you stand, sit down, or speak.

The predominant component of Meditation is to manage your thoughts. As you meditate and come to be more meditative, you will be able to manage your thoughts better than ever before. If you don't understand how to hold the mind and control your thoughts, it will put you thru all sorts of misery. If you allow the mind to be in charge, it is a horrible master.

Teachers and practitioners have also experienced the many physical and intellectual advantages of Meditation and yoga.

1. Meditation lowers excessive blood pressure and reduces stress. Actually, stress reduction is one of the most common motives humans strive for Meditation.
2. Controls Anxiety.
3. Promotes emotional health.
4. Enhances self-awareness.
5. Lengthens attention span.
6. Lowers the ranges of blood lactate, reducing anxiety attacks.
7. Serotonin production will increase to improve your mood. As you gain internal energy your immune system will also be developed.

As soon as you are in a meditative state, you are in the space of calmness, vastness, and joy.

Meditation can bring a real personal transformation. You'll naturally begin discovering more about yourself.

CHAPTER XIII
YOGA

♦ ♦ ♦

Health benefits of yoga are supported through science. Typical yoga is an ancient practice that brings together the mind and body. It contains breathing exercises, meditation, and poses designed to motivate relaxation and decrease stress. Multiple types of research have proven that it can limit the secretion of cortisol, the primary stress hormone. It can help you to lower your blood pressure which will reduce the risk of many problems.

One study has proven the powerful impact of yoga on stress through following 25 girls who perceived themselves as emotionally distressed. After a three-month yoga program, the girls had substantially decreased levels of cortisol. They additionally had decrease levels of stress, anxiety, fatigue, and depression. Another study of 135 people had comparable results, showing that 11 weeks of yoga helped enhance the quality of life and mental health.

Some studies advocate that practicing yoga may also decrease inflammation, as well. Inflammation is a natural immune response, but persistent inflammation can contribute to the development of diseases, such as heart disease, diabetes, and cancer.

In 2014 study divided 218 individuals into two groups, those who practiced yoga regularly and those who didn't both groups then performed moderate and strenuous workouts to result in stress.

At the end of the study, the people who practiced yoga had lower levels of inflammatory markers than those who didn't.

Similarly, in 2015 study confirmed that 12 weeks of yoga reduced inflammatory markers in breast cancer.

Yoga could Improve Heart Health.

From pumping blood throughout the body to providing tissues with vital nutrients, the health of your heart is a crucial element of overall health. Studies show that yoga may also enhance heart health and reduce the number of risk factors for heart disease, problems such as heart attacks and stroke.

One study discovered that participants over 35 years of age who practiced yoga for three years had lowered blood pressure and pulse rate.

A study observed 113 patients with heart disease, looking at the effects of a lifestyle change that included one year of yoga coaching combined with dietary adjustments and stress management. Participants noticed a 22% reduction in total cholesterol and a 27% reduction in (bad) LDL cholesterol. Additionally, the development of heart disease stopped in 48% of patients.

Yoga is becoming increasingly popular as a therapy to enhance the quality of life for many individuals.

Other research has looked at how yoga can improve the quality of life and decrease signs in patients with cancer. The study followed ladies with breast cancer undergoing chemotherapy had reduced symptoms of chemotherapy, such as nausea and vomiting, whilst additionally improving universal quality of life.

Many people add yoga to their fitness activities to improve flexibility and balance. It can optimize performance via the use of particular poses that target flexibility and balance.

A current study looked at the impact of 10 weeks of yoga on 28 male college athletes, practicing yoga considerably improved flexibility and balance. Practicing yoga could also help improve balance and mobility in older adults.

Practicing just 15–30 minutes of yoga every day could make a massive difference to enhance overall performance. It could help improve breathing.

Pranayama, or yogic breathing, is an exercise in yoga that focuses on controlling the breath via breathing exercises and techniques. Most kinds of yoga include these breathing exercises, and researchers have discovered that practicing yoga could help improve vital capacity. The essential capacity in amount of air person can expel from the lungs after a maximum inhalation. Increase in vital capacity will increase energy production. This is beneficial to the performance of an athlete especially crucial for those with lung disease, heart troubles, and asthma.

Based on these findings, practicing yoga can be a fantastic way to improve strength and endurance, mainly when used in combination with a regular exercise routine.

Multiple studies have confirmed the many mental and physical advantages of yoga.

Incorporating it into your routine can assist enhance your health, increase energy and flexibility, and reduce signs and symptoms of stress, depression, and anxiety. Practice yoga just a few times per week may be enough to make a significant difference when it comes to your health.

Virtual yoga classes are more advanced than ever, besides the many yoga DVDs and books on the market, on-line yoga lessons, and digital downloads are bringing home more of the benefits of live classes. While a teacher isn't always physically there to look at your alignment and regulate your pose hands-on, but still multimedia is the next fantastic thing, and for some, it may additionally be even better. You don't need much to begin home exercise. Choose or create a quiet, uncluttered area in your home for your practice, and stock it with the necessary simple yoga props mat, strap, blocks, blanket, bolster, etc. The place doesn't have to be big, but it must be quiet, clean, open, and sacred.

Begin with basic beginner's yoga sequences 10 to 15 minutes at a time and expand your exercise as your skills improve.

It's your yoga exercise, so build it to meet your personal needs best. Some of us like to do energizing yoga practice in the morning and a calming restorative practice in the evening.

When you practice your first poses on your own, try to cultivate a mindset of playfulness and acceptance try to be mindful. Being present during your exercise means allowing yourself to be aware of whatever physical sensations, emotions, and thoughts are currently arising. Be innovative and spontaneous. If you approach your practice with an experience of curiosity, rather than self-judgment or competitiveness, you will find it easier to encourage yourself to exercise.

As you advance, you may choose to move into more challenging intermediate and advanced yoga poses such as arm balances, inversions, and backbends.

CHAPTER XIV
EASY & HEALTHY RECIPES

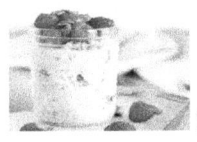 **Strawberry Overnight Jar 1.**

Serves 2 / preparing time 6 Mins / Ready in Overnight.

Ingredients:

1 ½ Cup oats

½ Cup of coconut yogurt

¼ Cup desiccated coconut

2 Tbsp. chia seeds

2 Tbsp. dried apricot

Toppings:

Strawberry / Strawberry puree / Pistachios / Additional coconut yoghurt / Fresh mint.

Method:

Mix 1 cup of oats and hot water in a large bowl cover it with a plate and leave it overnight.

In the morning divide between two jars (500ml) add a layer of 2 tbsp chia seeds, 2 tbsp dried apricot. Top with strawberry / Strawberry puree, pistachios, coconut yogurt, and fresh mint.

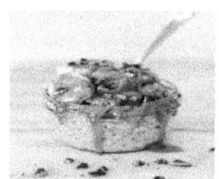

Mix Overnight Jar 2.

Ingredients:

1 Cup oats.

1 Tbsp, Pumpkin Seed.

1 Tbsp, peanut or almonds butter.

1 Tbsp, Walnuts.

1 Tbsp, Raw organic honey.

Method:

Mix 1 cup of oats and hot water in a large bowl cover it with a plate and leave it overnight.

In the morning, use tbsp to move oats into the glass jar, add a layer of pumpkin seeds and walnuts, leave a small place on top.

Add 1 tbsp, Almonds butter, 1 tbsp, raw organic honey, and enjoy. Or you can cover it and take it at work, but remember to keep it in the fridge.

AJAPSANDALI GEORGIAN EGGPLANT STEW.

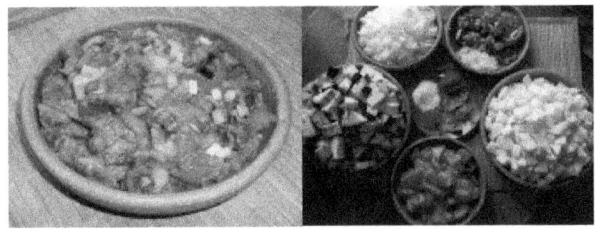

Ingredients: (serving five): 500 grams of potatoes, 600 grams of aubergine, 2 large tomatoes, 2 medium size onions, 3/4 green onions, 4 bay leaves, 3 green peppers, 2 red sweet peppers, 4 cloves of garlic, pinch of coriander, pinch of pink floor pepper, pinch of black ground pepper, a pinch of salt and 8 tsp of olive oil.

Preparation: Peel potatoes and chop all vegetables Add 5 tablespoons of water.

Put the chopped potatoes into a large pan, add chopped onion, chopped eggplant, three-bay leaves, and oil. Cover the pan and cook dinner on medium heat, stirring several instances till the veggies are cooked.

Remove the lid, add chopped tomatoes Stir and re-cover. After two minutes, add the chopped green and red peppers, garlic, coriander, red and black pepper, and salt. Stir, re-cover and cook dinner for a further 3 minutes.

Add some chopped green onions and enjoy your delicious Ajapsandali.

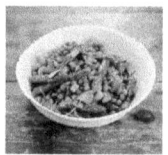

Pods & sods with watercress.

Ingredients:

A handful of asparagus, woody ends removed, each spear sliced into 4 pieces on an angle.

100/150 grams of fresh or frozen podded broad beans, better skins removed, 100/150 grams of fresh or frozen peas.

Sliced spring onions, 100g of watercress, 50g Alfalfa & Radish Sprouts for the dressing

4 Tbsp olive oil

5 Tsp white wine vinegar

Method:

Boil a large pan of water. Drop in the asparagus, wait to bring to the boil, and then add all the beans, and peas. Wait to bring back to the boil again, then you can drain and cool.

To make the dressing, mix the oil, vinegar, and some seasoning on the large platter, mix all the vegetables with the mint, spring onion, watercress, alfalfa & radish sprouts, and splash of the dressing.

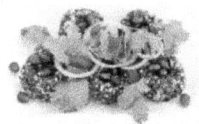 **Georgian spinach with walnuts.**

Ingredients:

2Pounds fresh spinach leaves.

1/2 Cups walnuts.

3Medium cloves garlic.

1Pack of fresh cilantro.

7Tablespoons of walnut oil or other flavored oil.

5Teaspoons tarragon vinegar or apple vinegar.

2Teaspoon ground coriander.

2Teaspoon kosher salt.

1Teaspoon ground fenugreek.

Several grinds of black pepper.

Pinch ground cayenne pepper.

1 Cup pomegranate seeds, for garnish.

Method:

Add spinach on to the boiled water, once all the spinach has softened, drain it in a large colander and rinse the spinach with tap water until the greens feel cool, then squeeze out the water by squeezing it as a chunk at a time, between your hands.

Transfer spinach in a large container, add ground walnuts, garlic, cilantro, oil, vinegar, coriander, salt, fenugreek, black pepper, and cayenne pepper. Adjust the seasonings as needed and mix them. Better keep in the refrigerator for 2/3 hours, or leave it overnight.

Add some pomegranate seeds, if using, just before serving.

Enjoy it as a spread on bread or on its own.

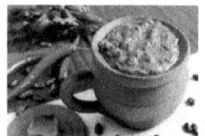

 Dry beans (Lobio) in a pot.

Ingredients:

3/4 Standard onions.

750 Grams of dry, red beans (Lobio).

2Bunches of clean coriander.

- Bunch of savory.
- Bunch of mints.
- Bunch of parsley.
- Bunch of celery.

4/5 Heads of garlic.

2/3 Leaves of bay-tree.

- Cooking Oil.
- Salt.
- Pepper.
- Vinegar or tkemali sauce.

Preparation:

Pour warm water onto the beans and boil, if the water evaporates, add more boiling water. When the beans are boiled, stir lightly (not to get puree), Chop some onions and fry them in olive oil. Then pour away the water and prepare the beans in a pot, add chopped herbs, garlic, fried onions, and tkemali sauce. The dish is now ready. Keep a small number of herbs apart to place on the beans when served at the table.

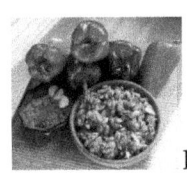

Red pepper stuffed with walnuts.

Ingredients:

Red bell pepper 6, Walnuts 160g, utskho suneli (fenugreek) 2 teaspoons, dried coriander 4 teaspoons, ground red pepper 1 teaspoon, 2/3 cloves of garlic, one onion, salt, pepper to taste, vinegar 2 tablespoons, olive oil 1 tablespoon.

Preparation:

Crush garlic and onion together with walnuts in the food

processor. Add some spices, 1 tablespoon of vinegar, 3-4 tablespoons of hot water and mix thoroughly until the mixture gets smooth. Remove the seeds form pepper. Boil the water, add salt, a tablespoon of oil, a tablespoon of vinegar, 1 bay leaf, and boil peppers for about 5 minutes. Take peppers out and cool, fill each pepper with walnuts paste using a spoon and put them on a plate. Place prepared peppers in the fridge for several hours so that all the flavors are blended well. Serve the dish cold. You can garnish red peppers with fresh chopped parsley as well. Enjoy it with whole-grain bread.

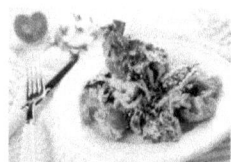

Cucumber-Tomato salad with walnuts.

Cucumber tomato salad with walnut dressing is a typical Georgian appetizer. The salad is served nearly at all Georgian restaurants, and it's very popular with tourists. The salad is made with fresh, delicious organic tomatoes, cucumbers and greens. The spicy walnut sauce is the main ingredient, which gives the dish its special flavor.

Ingredients:

3 tomatoes, 3 small cucumbers, 1 scallion or red onion, a handful of walnuts, 1 garlic clove, 1/2 tsp green chopped pepper, 1 tbsp red wine vinegar, few springs of cilantro and red basil, 1/2 cup water, Salt.

Preparation :

Put sliced cucumbers and tomatoes in a large bowl. In a food processor ground walnuts, garlic, cilantro, salt, add vinegar and water to thin the paste, and then pour it over the salad and mix it well if you like. To top it off, decorate with scallions and slightly chopped red basil.

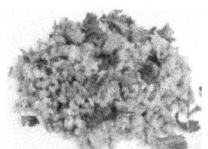

Using Cooked Buckwheat.

In case you have roasted buckwheat you don't even have to cook! To 100g of Buckwheat add 250ml of boiled water and leave it overnight and it will be ready to enjoy in the morning.

Buckwheat is a grain-like seed that's packed with vitamins and minerals like iron, magnesium, protein, essential amino acids, and more. The easiest way to prepare in case its roasted just add boiled water and leave it overnight, or you can cook buckwheat by boiling it like rice, and from there you can eat it on its own, serve it with meat, fish or even add fruit, vegetables and spices to make a tasty breakfast. There are also lots of different things you can do with buckwheat, which include making burgers, making a batch of granola, or even using the flour in baked goods.

1. Enjoy it on its own. Plain buckwheat is delicious and nutritious all by itself, either as a simple meal or as a side dish. To spice up plain cooked buckwheat, think about adding your favored herbs, spices, and seasonings, such as salt and pepper, Garlic or onion powder, Cumin, Cardamom, Fresh herbs such as parsley or cilantro.

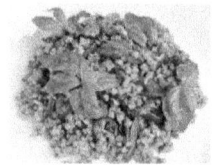

2. Stir fry it with vegetables.

Heat 1 tablespoon (16 ml) of cooking oil in a large frying pan. Cut 5 bell peppers into strips and put on the pan. Stir fry the peppers for about 4 minutes, add 6 cloves of minced garlic and 1 bunch of chopped kale. Cook the combination for another 5 minutes. Add the cooked buckwheat and 2 tablespoons (30 ml) of oil. Stir to mix all ingredients.

Before serving, garnish the stir fry with salt and pepper, to taste, add marinated artichoke hearts, and a handful of chopped basil if you like.

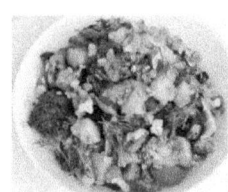

3. Cool it and toss it into a salad.

Set the cooked buckwheat aside to cool for about 25 minutes, and then transfer it to the refrigerator to chill for another 25 minutes. Once buckwheat is cold, mix it together in a bowl with any of your favorite vegetables and a simple dressing. As a sample salad recipe, to combine in a large bowl:

1 Medium cucumber, diced.

13 Olives, sliced.

1 Small bell pepper, diced.

1   Medium head of chopped broccoli florets.

1   Small onion, sliced thinly.

A handful of chopped almonds or walnuts.

½ Cup (13.5 g) fresh dill, minced.

1/2 Tablespoons (2/3 g) fresh mint, minced.

2/3 Tablespoons (35 ml) fresh lime juice.

2/3 Tablespoons (35 ml) wine vinegar.

1/2 Tablespoon (25 ml) olive oil.

Salt and pepper, to taste.

4. **You can make a breakfast meal by including fruit.**

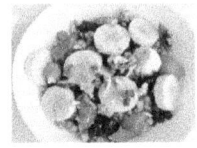

Transfer the cooked buckwheat to a saucepan and add 1 cup (236 ml) of dairy, almond or coconut milk. Bring the combination to a boil and remove the pan from the heat. Add 2 tablespoons (30 ml) of raw honey, 1 teaspoon (4.6 ml) of vanilla, and a pinch of ginger, cinnamon, nutmeg, or any different spices if you like. You can additionally top the porridge with fruit and nuts, such as:

Raspberries or blueberries, strawberries, sliced banana, raisins, dried currants, nut butter, chopped almonds, pistachios, or walnut.

CHAPTER XV
THE RAW FOOD DIET

❖ ❖ ❖

The raw food diet usually includes unprocessed, whole, plant-based, and ideally, organic foods. Three-quarters of the person's food plan must consist of uncooked food.

I believe that consuming a high percentage of uncooked meals makes you healthier.

Some raw foodists are vegan, and they eat no ingredients of animal origin. Others consume uncooked meat and raw animal products.

Weight loss is not the primary goal of the raw food diet. However, it is possible.

We know different types of raw food diets.

Raw vegetarians consume plant-based foods, plus eggs and dairy products. Of course, raw vegans consume no animal products at all.

Raw omnivores consume both plant-based and animal-based foods. All of these people generally consume raw food. A raw carnivore eats meat however not cooked meat.

What can I eat?

Suitable for the raw food diet:

Soaked beans, grains, dried fruits, raw nut butter, fresh fruits and uncooked vegetables, fruit and vegetable juices, milk from a young coconut, nut milk, raw nuts and seeds, purified water, but not tap water, seaweeds, sun-dried fruits, other organic, natural, or unprocessed foods, fermented foods, such as kimchi and sauerkraut.

Foods to avoid:

Milk and dairy products. Meat. Fish, for example, sushi or sashimi. Eggs. Refined sugars. Refined flour. Pasta, processed oils, table salt. All processed and cooked food.

Some of the raw foodists do eat fresh olives; however, not everyone because raw olives are bitter. Olives could be uncooked and sun-cured. Olives in cans are often cooked.

Different people have different interpretations of the uncooked meals, weight-reduction plan and what it means. Some people will eat some cooked food, while others eat none. However it depends on the people; for some people, it is a way of life. For others, it is a dietary choice.

Preparing the food:

A raw foodist makes food in a specific way by heating with a dehydrator, to blow hot air through the food. The temperature shouldn't be above 116 Fahrenheit or forty-six degrees Celsius. Raw foodists also may additionally mixture and chop up their foods. Beans seeds and grains can be eaten soaked.

Sample foods including:

Breakfast: Overnight soaked oats add nuts and fruits.

Lunch: Avocado salad. Apple and nut salad. Buckwheat salad.

Dinner: Pumpkin seed garlic pasta. Cauliflower rice with fresh peas.

Snack: Raw chocolate and coconut milk ice cream. Smoothie. Raw apple cinnamon chia bowl.

CHAPTER XVI
FOODS THAT BENEFIT VARIOUS BODY PARTS

♦ ♦ ♦

Food for Hair: 1, the protein is a primary source of hair, make sure you have enough protein to make your hair strong and healthy. 2, Iron is an exceptionally essential mineral for hair, and too little iron is a significant cause of hair loss. 3, Vitamin C aids the absorption of iron, so foods high in vitamin C are good to eat in conjunction with iron-rich foods. Vitamin C additionally increases collagen production in the body, which improves hair health. 4, Omega-3s oil keeps your scalp and hair hydrated. 5, Vitamin A is needed by the body to make something called sebum. The sebum is an oily substance created by our hairs sebaceous glands, and it supplies natural conditioning for a healthier scalp. Lack of sebum could lead to an itchy scalp and dry hair. 6, zinc plays a vital role in hair tissue growth and also repair; zinc deficiency can cause hair loss and a dry, flaky scalp. 7, Vitamin E is an antioxidant which can prevent oxidative stress and increase hair growth, it can also help your skin and hair from sun damage, so ensure you eat foods rich in vitamin E. 8, Biotin plays an essential role in hair growth. Your body doesn't store biotin, so regular intake of biotin is necessary. The lack of biotin can also lead to hair loss, dry skin, and eyes.

1. **Protein:** Chicken, turkey, fish, dairy products, eggs, legumes, nuts.
2. **Iron:** lentils, spinach, broccoli, kale, salad greens.
3. **Vitamin C:** blackcurrants, blueberries, broccoli, guava, kiwi fruits, oranges, papaya, strawberries, sweet potatoes.
4. **Omega-3s:** salmon, herring, sardines, trout, mackerel, avocado, pumpkin seeds, walnuts.
5. **Vitamin A:** Cheese, eggs, oily fish, fortified low-fat spreads, carrots, pumpkins, and sweet potatoes.
6. **Zinc and selenium:** cereals, whole grains, oysters, beef, and eggs.
7. **Vitamin E:** Sunflower seeds, almonds, hazelnuts, pine nuts, peanuts, brazil nuts, pistachios, pumpkin seeds.
8. **Biotin:** Liver, yeast, egg yolk, milk, cheese, yogurt, avocado, sweet potato, cauliflower.

Natural treatments:

Make your very own hair masks for a deep, nourishing cure every two weeks. Whisk an egg yolk and combine with 1 tbsp of honey and more than half of mashed avocado. Massage onto moistured, clean hair and leave for 25 minutes before rinsing thoroughly.

Food for Skin: Red peppers, brussel sprouts, lemons, oranges, grapefruits, blueberries, sweet potatoes, cottage cheese, carrots, mango, edamame, tomatoes, brown rice, salmon, pumpkin seeds.

Food for Eyes: Egg yolks, yellow corn.

Food for Brain: Salmon, tuna, sardines, turmeric, broccoli, pumpkin seeds, dark chocolate, oranges.

Food for Bones: Milk, fortified soy beverages, kale, collards, tofu, pumpkin seeds, almonds.

Food for Heart: Baked potato, prune juice, avocado, berries, fatty fish and fish oil, beans, walnuts, dark chocolate.

Food for Lungs: Broccoli, brussels sprouts, bok choy.

Food for Stomach: Ginger, mint, papaya, fennel, chamomile tea.

Food for Colon: Beans and peas, kale, spinach, chard, and raspberries.

Food for Prostate: Green tea, berries, salmon, nuts.

Food for Ovaries: spinach, broccoli, turmeric, and tomatoes.

Food for kidneys: Apples, berries, dark leafy greens, sweet potatoes, fatty fish, water.

Food for the urinary system: Berries, yogurt, garlic, apples, grapes, peanuts, and cinnamon.

Food for men's reproductive system: Oysters, crab, lobster, nuts and beans, ginseng root, maca root, ashwagandha root.

Food for the gut: Sauerkraut, tempeh, kimchi, miso, kefir, broccoli, asparagus, seaweed, green apples, banana, Jerusalem artichoke, and flaxseed.

Food for pancreas: Beans and lentils, flax, milk and almond milk, spinach, blueberries, cherries, whole grains.

Food for liver: Coffee, grapefruit, blueberries and cranberries, grapes, pear, nuts, Beetroot juice, olive oil, Fatty fish.

Food for thymus: Thymus is a small gland that lies behind the breast bone between the lungs. One of the main functions of the thymus is to produce immune system cells that fight diseases like cancer, but the problem is that thymus shrinks rapidly with age, reducing the ability of older people to respond to new challenges to their immune system. The cells are unendingly lost and replaced throughout life. However, many of vitamin C rich foods like dark leafy greens, Brussels sprouts, oranges, tomatoes, kiwi fruit, berries, and broccoli, protect the thymus gland, a vital immune system organ. Fruits like papaya, strawberries, pineapple, cantaloupe, raspberries, cranberries, blueberries, and watermelon are also excellent sources of vitamin C.

Food for thyroid gland: Iodized table salt, spinach, lettuce, cashews, almonds, pumpkin seeds, Brazil nuts, fish, shrimp, seaweed.

CHAPTER XVII
ESSENTIAL VITAMINS AND MINERALS
♦ ♦ ♦

Vitamins and minerals are considered essential nutrients your body needs in small quantities to work correctly and stay healthy. Most people need to get all the vitamins they need using a varied and balanced diet, although some people might also need to take extra supplements. Vitamins and minerals are as essential for your body as air and water. Not only do they maintain your body healthy and functional, but they also defend you from a range of diseases.

Vitamins and minerals get thrown together. However, they are pretty different. Vitamins are organic components produced via plants or animals. They often are known as essential due to the fact they are not synthesized in the body "except for vitamin D" and therefore need to come from the food we eat daily.

Minerals are a chemical compound that is formatted naturally on the earth. Originate from soil, rocks, or water. But you can absorb them indirectly from the environment or an animal that has eaten a specific plant.

Vitamins are divided into two classes: water-soluble, which means the body expels what it does not absorb and fat-soluble where remaining amounts are saved in the liver and fat tissues as reserves. The water-soluble vitamins are the eight B vitamins (B-1, B-2, B-3, B-5, B-6, B-7, B-9, and B-12) and vitamin C, and the fat-soluble vitamins are A, D, E, and K.

There are many minerals. However, certain ones are vital for optimum health. Minerals are split into two main groups: major and trace. Major ones are not necessarily more essential than a trace. However, it means there are higher amounts in your body.

The best strategy to make sure you get a range of vitamins and minerals, and in the desired amounts, is to adopt a comprehensive healthy diet, this includes an emphasis on fruits and vegetables, whole grains, beans and legumes, low-fat protein, and dairy products. The good news is that many everyday meals contain more than one mineral and vitamin sources, so it is effortless to meet your daily needs from daily meals.

Vitamins and minerals, their functions, and food sources:

Vitamin A.

Vitamin A has several essential functions these include: helping your body's natural defense against illness and infection (the immune system) helping vision in dim light, keeping skin healthy.

Some of the best sources of vitamin A are yellow vegetables and fruits, such as orange. Eggs, oily fish, cheese, fortified low-fat spreads, milk, and yogurt.

The amount of vitamin A adults aged 18 to 65 need is 0.7mg a day for men and 0.6mg a day for women.

Vitamin B.

There are eight types of vitamin B.

Thiamin (vitamin B1)

Riboflavin (vitamin B2)

Niacin (vitamin B3)

Pantothenic acid (vitamin B5)

Pyridoxine (vitamin B6)

Biotin (vitamin B7)

Folate and folic acid (vitamin B9)

Cobalamin (vitamin B12)

Thiamin, also known as vitamin B1, helps:

Break down and release energy from food. Keep the nervous system healthy. Some sources of thiamin include:

Fresh, dried fruit, eggs, peas, wholegrain bread, and some fortified breakfast cereals.

The amount of thiamin adults (aged 18 to 65) need is: 1mg a day for men and 0.8mg a day for women.

Vitamin B2.

Vitamin B2, riboflavin is essential for our health. It helps the body break down carbohydrates, Keep eyes, skin, and the nervous system healthy.

Some sources of riboflavin include eggs, milk, rice, fortified breakfast cereals. The problem is that UV light can destroy riboflavin, so ideally, these foods should be kept out of direct sunlight.

The amount of riboflavin adults (aged 18 to 65) need is about:

1.3mg a day for men and 1.1mg a day for women.

Vitamin B3 niacin.

Vitamin B3, also called niacin, has a wide range of benefits for the body. It helps release energy from the foods we eat, keep the nervous system, and skin healthy. We know that there are two forms of niacin: nicotinic acid and nicotinamide. Both are found in food. Some sources of niacin include meat, fish, wheat flour, eggs, and milk. The amount of niacin adult need is about: 16 mg a day for men and 14 mg a day for women.

Pantothenic acid vitamin B5.

Pantothenic acid has numerous functions, such as supporting to release energy from food, making blood cells.

Some sources of pantothenic acid include beef, chicken, porridge, potatoes, tomatoes, kidney, eggs, broccoli, brown rice, and whole meal bread.

We should be able to get all the pantothenic acid we need from our daily diet, as it is discovered in foods that are good sources of vitamin B. However, the body can't store pantothenic acid, so you need it in your diet every day.

Pyridoxine-Vitamin B6.

Vitamin B6 is needed for brain development. It helps the body make serotonin that regulates mood, and norepinephrine which helps to cope with stress.

Some sources of vitamin B6 include Wholegrain cereals, poultry such as chicken or turkey, pork, fish, bread, vegetables, eggs, peanuts, milk, potatoes, and some fortified breakfast cereals.

The quantity of vitamin B6 adults (aged 18 to 65) need is about:

1.4mg a day for men and 1.2mg a day for women.

Biotin (vitamin B7).

Biotin is needed in tiny quantities to help the body break down fat. The microorganism that lives naturally in your bowel is capable of making biotin. Biotin is additionally found in a wide range of foods but at very low levels. In case you take biotin supplements, make sure you do not exceed the recommended dose, as this could be harmful for your health. An adult needs no more than 0.9mg of biotin a day.

Folate and folic acid - Vitamin B9.

Folate is a B vitamin discovered small quantities in many different foods. Folate is called folic acid, folacin, and vitamin B9.

Folate helps the body form healthy red blood cells; it reduces the risk of anemia and high blood pressure, helps pregnant women reduce the risk of birth defects. We should try to avoid a lack of folate as it could lead to folate deficiency anemia.

Some sources of folate include broccoli, brussel sprouts, liver but keep away from the liver during pregnancy! cabbage, spinach, peas, chickpeas, breakfast cereals fortified with folic acid.

An adult person needs 200 micrograms of folate a day. The word microgram is occasionally written with the Greek image μ, followed by the letter g (μg). However, the body can't store folate in the long-term, so we have to eat folate-containing foods from time to time.

If in case you are pregnant or trying for a baby, it's good to have 400 micrograms of folic acid supplement each day till you are 12 weeks pregnant, it will prevent birth defects such as spinal Bifida in the baby. In any case, I would recommend speaking to your doctor about it during the pregnancy.

Vitamin B12.

Vitamin B12 is associated with making red blood cells and keeping the nervous system healthy. We need to get enough B12 because a lack of vitamin B12 could lead to vitamin B12 deficiency anemia.

Some sources of vitamin B12 include meat, salmon, cod, milk, cheese, eggs, and some fortified breakfast cereals.

Adults (aged 18 to 65) need about 1.5 micrograms a day of vitamin B12. If we eat meat, fish, or dairy foods, we should be able to get enough vitamin B12. Vegans can get enough vitamin B12 from food fortified with B12, or they have to take supplements.

Vitamin C.

Vitamin C is additionally known as ascorbic acid. Vitamin C has many important functions in our body. These include: Formation of collagen, immune system, wound healing, helping to protect cells, maintaining healthy skin, bones, and cartilage.

Make sure you have enough Vitamin C because the lack of vitamin C can lead to scurvy.

Sources of vitamin C include red and green peppers, oranges, strawberries, blackcurrants, broccoli, Brussel sprouts, and potatoes.

Adults aged 18 to 65 need 40mg of vitamin C a day.

Vitamin D.

Vitamin D helps absorb calcium; it helps to build bones and to keep teeth strong and healthy.

In case you don't get enough of vitamin D can lead to bone and back pain, rickets in children. The sun is a very good source of vitamin D: From late march to the end of September; most people should be in a position to get enough vitamin D they need from sunlight. But it depends where you live, between October and early March we don't get enough vitamin D from sunlight. Vitamin D is additionally discovered in a small variety of foods such as salmon, sardines, herring, mackerel, red meat, liver, and egg yolks.

Usually, children from the age of 12 months, and adults need ten micrograms of vitamin D a day.

Vitamin E.

Vitamin E acts as an antioxidant; it helps prevent coronary heart diseases; it helps maintain healthy skin and healthy eyes, helping to protect cells from the damage, strengthens the body's natural defense against illness and infection. Some sources of vitamin E include Corn and olive oil, nuts, and seeds.

The adult person needs around 14mg vitamin E a day.

If there is a vitamin E your body doesn't need, it will be stored for future use, so you don't have to eat vitamin E rich food every day.

Vitamin K.

Vitamin K is essential for human health; it plays an important role in blood clotting and bone metabolism. It helps wounds heal properly and help maintain bones healthy. Vitamin K is found in spinach, broccoli, kale, collards, and parsley.

Adults need approximately one microgram of vitamin K a day for each kilogram of their body weight. For example, anyone who weighs 60kg would need 60 micrograms a day of vitamin K, while an individual who weighs 70kg would need 70 micrograms a day.

Calcium.

Calcium has numerous essential functions, and these include: Helping build strong bones and teeth. It's necessary for muscle contractions, which includes your heartbeat. It plays an important part in the blood clotting process.

If your body doesn't get enough calcium, it could lead to

RICKETS in children, and OSTEOMALACIA or OSTEOPOROSIS in later life.

Sources of calcium include milk, cheese, broccoli, cabbage, okra: tofu, nuts, bread, and the fish where you eat the bones.

Adults aged 18 to 65 need 700mg of calcium a day. We shouldn't take excessive doses of calcium. More than 1,500mg a day could lead to belly pain and diarrhea.

Iodine.

Iodine helps make thyroid hormones, which help preserve cells and the metabolic rate. Some food sources of iodine include: Seaweed, sea fish, shellfish.

Adults 14 years old and over need 0.15mg of iodine a day.

Taking excessive doses of iodine for long periods of time could be harmful. It could have an effect on your thyroid gland and lead to a wide range of different symptoms, such as eosinophilia, fever, headache, and weight gain.

Iron.

The lack of iron can lead to iron-deficiency anemia. The iron is important for making red blood cells that carries oxygen around the body. Some sources of iron include liver "but keep away from this during pregnancy" beans, nuts and dried apricots, meat, brown rice, soybean flour, watercress, and curly kale.

The amount of iron we need is: Male 14–18 years 10 mg female 14 mg or 26 mg if you are pregnant. Male 18-55 years 9 mg, female 17 mg. 50+ years old both male and female 9 mg. Women who lose a lot of blood throughout their monthly period "heavy periods" are at greater chance of iron deficiency anemia and may need to take iron supplements. Speak to your doctor or a registered dietitian for more advice.

Side effects of taking excessive doses (over 20mg) of iron include: Constipation, feeling sick, vomiting, stomach pain.

Excessive doses of iron can be fatal, especially for children, so always keep iron supplements out of the reach of children.

A healthy diet includes many other nutrients as well as common minerals and vitamins such as chromium, beta-carotene, cobalt, copper, magnesium, manganese molybdenum, phosphorus, potassium, selenium, salt, and zinc.

Beta-carotene.

Beta-carotene gives its yellow color to fruit and vegetables. It will turn into vitamin A in the body so that it can perform the same jobs in the body as vitamin A.

The main sources of beta-carotene are Sweet potato, spinach, carrots, red peppers, mango, papaya, apricots, and winter squash.

Chromium.

Chromium is thought to have an effect on how the hormone insulin behaves in the body. Chromium supplements also could be helpful for people with type 2 diabetes.

Some sources of chromium include meat, whole meal bread, and whole oats, lentils, broccoli, potatoes, and spices.

Up to 25 micrograms of chromium a day should be sufficient for adults.

Cobalt.

Cobalt makes up part of vitamin B12. Some sources of cobalt include fish, nuts, broccoli, spinach, and oats.

In case you get enough vitamin B12, you'll also get enough cobalt.

Having excessive amounts of cobalt for lengthy periods of time may affect the heart and would possibly decrease fertility in men.

Copper.

Copper is an essential nutrient that has an important role in our body, together with iron, it produces red blood cells. It's additionally thought to be important for baby growth, brain development, the immune system, and strong bones.

Some sources of copper include nuts, shellfish, and offal.

Adult aged 18 to 65 needs 1.2mg of copper a day.

Taking excessive doses of copper could cause Stomach pain, sickness, and diarrhea. If we take it for long periods, it could damage the liver and kidneys.

Magnesium.

Magnesium is a very important mineral because it regulates muscle function, including the heart muscle; it also regulates blood pressure and the production of cholesterol, helps parathyroid glands, which produce hormones essential for bone health, to work normally.

The source of magnesium: Spinach, nuts, brown rice, whole grain bread, fish, meat, dairy foods.

The amount of magnesium we need is: 300mg a day for men (18 to 65 years) and 270mg a day for women (18 to 65 years)

Taking excessive doses of magnesium (more than 400mg) can cause digestive issues and diarrhea.

Manganese.

Manganese is important for our health because it is a key component of some enzymes. It supports brain function.

Manganese has been discovered in a wide variety of foods, including bread, tea nuts, cereals, peas, and runner beans.

Taking high doses of manganese may cause muscle pain, nerve damage, and different symptoms, such as fatigue and depression.

Molybdenum.

Molybdenum is an essential mineral found in legumes and grains. Molybdenum helps to remove toxins from the metabolism of sulfur-containing amino acids.

Some of the richest sources of molybdenum include Lentils, beans, oats, peas, broccoli, spinach, and cauliflower.

Phosphorus.

Phosphorus is very important because it helps build strong bones and teeth; it helps release energy from food.

Some richest sources of phosphorus include Red meat, dairy foods, fish, poultry, bread, brown rice, and oats.

Adults need 550mg of phosphorus a day.

Taking excessive doses of phosphorus supplements can be toxic; it can cause diarrhea or hardening of organs and soft tissues, which can decrease the amount of calcium in the body, which means bones are more likely to fracture, can affect body's ability to use of iron, magnesium, and zinc effectively.

Potassium.

Potassium is an essential mineral for the human body, and it helps control the balance of fluids in the body and additionally supports the heart muscle to work correctly.

Some sources of potassium include: Bananas, broccoli, parsnips, brussels sprouts, pulses, nuts, seeds, fish, shellfish, beef, chicken, and turkey.

Adults (18 to 65 years) need 3,500mg of potassium a day. We must be in a position to get all the potassium we need from our daily diet.

Taking too much potassium can cause belly pain, feeling sick, and diarrhea.

Selenium.

Selenium plays an important role in health; it helps the immune system work properly. It additionally helps prevent damage of cells and tissues.

Some sources of selenium include: Brazil nuts, fish, meat, eggs, and mushrooms.

The amount of selenium you need is:

0.075mg a day for men 18 to 65 years.

0.06mg a day for ladies 18 to 65 years.

If you eat Brazil nuts, mushrooms, meat, or fish, you should be able to get enough selenium your body needs.

Make sure you don't exceed the recommended dose because too much selenium can cause selenosis, the condition that could be very harmful because it leads to loss of hair, skin, and nails.

Sodium chloride (salt).

Sodium chloride is typically known as salt.

Sodium and chloride are minerals needed by our body in small quantities to assist and maintain the level of fluids in the body, but too little or too much salt can be harmful to our health. Chloride additionally helps the body digest food.

Usually, salt is found at low levels in all foods, but some salt is added to many processed foods, such as: Chips, meat products, ready meals, some breakfast cereals, cheese, some bread, savory snacks.

We don't need more than 6g of salt (2.4g of sodium) a day. But, on average, people consume 8g of salt (about 3.2g of sodium) a day, which is a lot more than the body needs.

I would suggest you check food labels and pick them with less salt. And where color-coded labels are used, try to choose products with more greens and ambers and fewer reds for a more healthy choice. In case you are buying tinned fish, choose in spring water instead of brine.

Try to avoid sauces – like soy sauce, brown sauce, ketchup, and mayonnaise. Eat fewer salty snacks, such as salted nuts and crisps — salty meats such as bacon, cheese, pickles, and smoked fish. When cooking, add less salt or no salt at all use herbs and spices for flavor instead. Taste your meals first, and don't mechanically add more.

Having too much salt will cause high blood pressure, which raises your risk of serious problems like strokes and heart attacks.

Zinc.

Zinc is a nutrient that plays a very important role in your body. Zinc helps make new cells, enzymatic reactions, wound healing, immune functions, growth, and development.

Some sources of zinc include meat, shellfish, cheese, bread, and cereal products.

The amount of zinc we need is about: 9.5mg a day for men and 7mg for women. Taking an excessive amount of zinc will reduce the amount of copper your body can absorb, and this could lead to anemia and weakening of the bones.

Vitamin and mineral sources in short.

Water-soluble:

B-1: Ham, soymilk, watermelon, acorn squash, Peas, Fresh and dried fruit, Eggs, Wholegrain bread, some fortified breakfast cereals.

B-2: Yogurt, cheese, milk, eggs, fortified breakfast cereals, rice.

B-3: Fish, wheat flour, eggs, milk, meat, poultry, fortified and whole grains, mushrooms, potatoes.

B-5: Chicken, beef, potatoes, porridge, tomatoes, kidney, eggs, broccoli, whole meal bread, brown rice, avocados, mushrooms.

B-6: Pork, poultry such as chicken or turkey, fish, bread, wholegrain cereals, such as oatmeal, wheat germ, and brown rice, vegetables, eggs, peanuts, milk, potatoes, legumes, tofu, bananas.

B-7: Whole grains, eggs, soybeans, fish.

B-9: Broccoli, Brussels sprouts, cabbage and spinach, peas, chickpeas, fortified grains and cereals, asparagus.

B-12: Meat, salmon, milk, cheese, eggs, some fortified breakfast cereals, poultry.

Vitamin - C: Oranges and orange juice, red and green peppers, strawberries, blackcurrants, broccoli, Brussel sprouts, potatoes, bell peppers, spinach, and tomatoes.

Fat-soluble:

Vitamin - A: Cheese, eggs, oily fish, fortified low-fat spreads, milk and yogurt, beef, liver, eggs, shrimp, sweet potatoes, carrots, pumpkins, spinach, mangoes.

Vitamin - D: Salmon, sardines, herring and mackerel, red meat, liver, egg yolks.

Vitamin - E: Corn and olive oil, nuts and seeds, leafy green vegetables, whole grains.

Vitamin - K: Broccoli and spinach, vegetable oils, cereal grains, cabbage, kale.

Minerals

Major:

Calcium: Milk, cheese, and different dairy foods, green leafy greens – such as broccoli, cabbage, and okra. Soya beans, tofu, nuts, bread, and whatever made with fortified flour, sardines, and pilchards.

Chloride: salt, ready meat, bacon, breakfast cereals, and Cheese.

Magnesium: Spinach, nuts, brown rice, whole grain bread, fish, meat, dairy foods, broccoli, legumes, seeds.

Potassium: Bananas, broccoli, parsnips, brussels sprouts, pulses, nuts and seeds, shellfish, beef, chicken, turkey.

Sodium: Salt, soy sauce, vegetables.

Trace:

Chromium: Fish, nuts, cheese, meat, whole meal bread and whole oats, lentils, broccoli, potatoes, spices, chicken, turkeys.

Copper: Seeds, nuts, whole grain products, shellfish, beans, prunes.

Fluoride: Fish, teas, fluoridated water.

Iodine: Seaweed, sea fish, shellfish, Iodized salt.

Iron: Meat, beans, nuts, dried fruit – such as dried apricots, whole grains, poultry, eggs, fruits, green vegetables, fortified bread.

Manganese: Tea, bread, nuts, cereals, peas, legumes, whole grains.

Selenium: Brazil nuts, fish, meat, eggs, mushrooms, seafood, walnuts.

Zinc: Meat, shellfish, cheese, bread, cereal products, legumes, whole grains.

Beta-carotene: Spinach, carrots and red peppers, mango, papaya, and apricots.

Copper: Oysters, nuts, seeds, shitake mushrooms, lobster, shellfish, offal.

Molybdenum: Nuts, tinned vegetables, cereals – such as oats, peas, broccoli, spinach, and cauliflower.

Phosphorus: Red meat, dairy foods, fish, poultry, bread, brown rice, oats.

Some of the best variety of foods you can include in your diet to receive all the necessary vitamins and minerals, without needing to take tablets, liquid form of minerals and vitamins unless doctor subscribes it:

Nuts:

Brazil nuts, almonds, walnuts, cashew nuts, peanuts, pecan nuts, pili nuts.

Fruits:

Banana, watermelon, orange, lemon, strawberries, grapefruit, blackberries, apples, pomegranate, pineapple, avocado, blueberries, peaches, grapes, kiwi, mangoes, raspberries, cranberries, tart cherries, papaya, okra, summer squash, winter squash, cantaloupe, cranberry, figs, grapefruit, pears, plums, mulberries, rose hip, cocoa powder, summer squash, raisins.

Bread and Grains:

Whole grains, whole wheat bread, buckwheat, brown rice, oats, quinoa.

Seeds:

Flaxseeds, sunflower seeds, pumpkin seeds, black pepper, cinnamon, peppermint.

Vegetable:

Broccoli, spinach, sweet potatoes, carrots, green peas,

asparagus, arugula, tomatoes, seaweed, garlic, brussels sprouts, swiss chard, ginger, cabbage, collard greens, onions, coriander, beet greens, beetroot, watercress, kale, red bell pepper, alfalfa sprouts, cucumber, artichokes, celery, mushrooms, bok choy, cauliflower, corn, eggplant, fennel, leeks, mustard greens, turnip greens, romaine lettuce, black beans, lentils, turmeric, Jerusalem artichoke.

Dairy: Organic cheese, grass-fed yogurt, organic cow milk.

Meat & Egg: Organic lean beef, lamb, chicken breast, turkey breast, organic eggs.

Fish: Salmon, tuna, oysters, sardines, shellfish, shrimp, trout, scallops.

Oils: Chia seed oil, pumpkin seed oil, extra virgin olive oil, black Seed oil, coconut oil.

Others: Apple cider vinegar, dark chocolate, raw honey, bee pollen, fermented food such as kefir, miso, sauerkraut, lassi, kimchi, tempeh, kombuch.

Listen to your body:

I have stated scientific truth to what and how much vitamins and minerals an adult person needs daily. However, the truth is that only our body knows what each need. Listening to your body is the key to determine how much and what you need to eat.

Your body knows what it wants. In order to keep running efficiently, it needs the fuel of vitamin and nutrient-rich meals from a range of food groups. If you listen to your body, it will tell you exactly what it needs. The 1st most crucial aspect of listening to your body is to be able to feel when you are getting hungry. If you are indeed starving, and what are the vitamins and minerals your body is asking, but not just looking for food to cure your boredom, stress, or loneliness. The 2nd key is being able to know when you have had enough. Listen to your body! When you begin to sense full, you will be aware that you have had enough to eat. The goal is to detect content not uncomfortably stuffed but not starving either. For some people, this means planning 4 or 5 smaller, well-balanced meals a day. And remember, it takes about 20 to 30 minutes for your body to realize it's full. Try to eat mindfully, be aware of what you are eating, make sure you sit down when you are eating, chew slowly, enjoy the tastes, and smells of your food. Learn about conscious or intuitive eating.

AESTHETICS

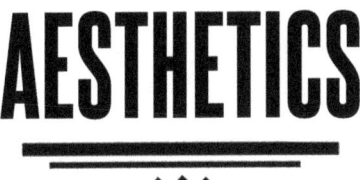

To conclude everything I have mentioned above:

1. Meditate.
2. Eat healthy. Try to adjust at least 70/80 percent of your daily diet from green pages.
3. Remove toxic and dishonest people from your life no matter if they are family, colleagues, or friends.
4. Don't chase after money, money will never make you happy; don't think it will give you a life of wealth and automatic happiness.
5. Don't tie yourself up in unnecessary contracts such as a gym membership, fancy mobile phone, etc.
6. Certainly don't take a mortgage in big cities where prices are inflated so much that you will be forced to pay it back in 25 to 30 years, but if you still do, be advised that you willingly sign up for life long slavery. Only take a mortgage if you can pay it back in 10 years max.

7. Big cities are the most polluted places to live, try to live in the countryside.
8. Exercise.
9. Have a social life.
10. Try to have a healthy, decent sex life.
11. Remember that you are going to die one day no matter what you own, so why would you enslave yourself, why would you sacrifice your limited life for something that doesn't make any sense at the end of the day.
12. Give to receive, yes that is right, but be careful, don't get robbed! You will receive the way you give. When you give don't look back. If you do, you are trading, so in this case you should expect your return from the individual or organization either as profit or loss, depending on whom you are trading with. If you reach a stage of giving unconditionally without looking back, losing your mind, and getting robbed, then you may receive accordingly.
13. Seek virtue, become virtuous.
14. Sleep. Make sure to get enough good sleep. Sleep puts you in a better mood, can help you maintain your weight, lowers your blood pressure, helps reduce stress, and improves your memory. Sleep helps keep your heart healthy.

More and less I have included everything that I consider as wise and helpful. Hopefully this will help you to live a healthier and happier life.

Lightning Source UK Ltd.
Milton Keynes UK
UKHW012049210622
404755UK00003B/293